Massage and Bodywork

Adapting Therapies for Cancer Care

Edited by

Peter A Mackereth

PhD, MA RGN, Cert Ed, Dip Nursing
Clinical Lead and Lecturer, Complementary
Therapies, Christie Hospital, Manchester and Salford
University, Greater Manchester, UK

Ann Carter

BA, Dip Health Ed, Cert Ed, MIFPA
Complementary Therapy Co-ordinator,
St Ann's Hospice, and Trainer in Complementary
Therapies, Manchester, UK

Forewords by

Denise Rankin-Box, BA (Hons), RGN, Dip TD, Cert Ed, MISMA, JP
Editor-in-Chief, Complementary Therapies in Clinical Practice

Michele Angelo Petrone, BA, Director of MAP Foundation, Honorary
Lecturer at Royal Free & University College London Medical School,
Senior Honorary Lecturer at University of Northumbria at Newcastle,
Professional artist and cancer patient

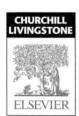

Edinburgh London New York Oxford Philadelphia St Louis
Sydney Toronto 2006

CHURCHILL
LIVINGSTONE
ELSEVIER

An imprint of Elsevier Limited

© Elsevier Ltd 2006

Churchill Livingstone is a registered trademark of Elsevier Limited

The right of Peter Mackereth and Ann Carter to be identified as the authors of this work has been asserted in accordance with the Copyright, Designs and Patents Act 1988.

First published 2006
ISBN-10: 0 443 10031 4
ISBN-13: 978 0 443 10031 4

British Library Cataloguing in Publication Data
A catalogue record for this book is available from the British Library

Library of Congress Cataloging in Publication Data
A catalogue record for this book is available from the Library of Congress

---

Notice

Knowledge and best practice in this field are constantly changing. As new research and experience broaden our knowledge, changes in practice, treatment and drug therapy may become necessary or appropriate. Readers are advised to check the most current information provided (i) on procedures featured or (ii) by the manufacturer of each product to be administered, to verify the recommended dose or formula, the method and duration of administration, and contraindications. It is the responsibility of the practitioner, relying on their own experience and knowledge of the patient, to make diagnoses, to determine dosages and the best treatment for each individual patient, and to take all appropriate safety precautions. To the fullest extent of the law, neither the publisher nor the editor assumes any liability for any injury and/or damage.

The Publisher

Working together to grow
libraries in developing countries
www.elsevier.com | www.bookaid.org | www.sabre.org

ELSEVIER   BOOK AID International   Sabre Foundation

ELSEVIER

your source for books,
journals and multimedia
in the health sciences
www.elsevierhealth.com

Printed in China
The Publisher's policy is to use paper manufactured from sustainable forests

Massage
and
Bodywork

For Elsevier:

Senior Commissioning Editor: Sarena Wolfaard
Development Editor: Kerry McGechie
Project Manager: Morven Dean
Design Direction: Judith Wright
Illustration Buyer: Merlyn Harvey
Illustrator: David Gardner

Contents

About the Editors

PETER A MACKERETH, PhD, MA RGN, Cert Ed, Dip Nursing, has occupied roles such as Intensive Care Charge Nurse, Nurse Consultant and Research Associate. Peter was awarded his PhD in October 2005. His research project was concerned with examining therapeutic outcomes for reflexology and relaxation. As a practising reflexologist, and massage and bodywork therapist, he works with patients in healthcare settings and private practice. Peter has published widely, speaks at conferences and lectures on academic programmes in the university sector.

ANN CARTER, BA, Dip Health Ed, Cert Ed, MIFPA, has qualifications in massage, aromatherapy and neurolinguistic programming. She has also studied CranioSacral Therapy™ and is a qualified Life Coach. Ann became involved in providing therapy for patients with cancer in 1994 when she joined the team at the Neil Cliffe Cancer Care Centre in Manchester. In 2000, Ann was appointed as Complementary Therapy Co-ordinator for the three sites of St Ann's Hospice. In addition she teaches on a range of under-graduate and post-graduate courses for therapists and healthcare professionals. She has designed and facilitated (with others) a course for complementary therapy co-ordinators and is Principal Tutor for the Complementary Therapy in Cancer Care Course at the Christie Hospital, Manchester.

Contributors

JILL BAILEY, MCSP, HPC registrant MRSS, works as Senior Lecturer in Physiotherapy at Manchester Metropolitan University. In addition to her role as physiotherapist, Jill is a shiatsu practitioner. She has experience as a clinical specialist physiotherapist and complementary therapy practitioner in both palliative care and mental healthcare within the NHS. Jill has established and co-ordinated a physiotherapy and complementary therapy service at the Trafford Macmillan Care Centre in Manchester, and uses shiatsu with patients in private practice.

GWYNNETH CAMPBELL, BA (Hons), PGCE, is a complementary therapy practitioner at the Christie Hospital where she leads a practice development project which provides chair massage to carers. Apart from her clinical work with patients, carers and staff, Gwynneth teaches a variety of courses related to complementary therapies and healthcare and she also facilitates group and individual clinical supervision for therapists. Gwynneth has a private practice offering therapeutic massage, Chiron healing and stress management.

JOANNE CARR, MCSP, SRP, is a Senior Physiotherapist, specialising in neurological care. Joanne has developed a spinal cord compression pathway involving the multidisciplinary team in cancer care and has also contributed to the National Institute for Health and Clinical Excellence (NICE) guidelines for improving outcomes in patients with central nervous system tumours. Joanne has registered for an MSc and has been working with June Rosen on the Spinal Cord Compression and Massage Project at Christie Hospital, Manchester.

ANNE CAWTHORN, MSc, BSc (Hons), Dip Nursing, RGN, OND, RNT, Ad TA Cert, is a Lecturer Practitioner at the Christie Hospital and Manchester University. She previously co-ordinated the complementary therapies at the Neil Cliffe Cancer Centre and St Ann's Hospice in Manchester. Her practice involves counselling and psychotherapy with patients and carers, and providing clinical supervision to healthcare professionals, including massage therapists.

BARBARA COOK, MAR, AoR, has completed training in aromatherapy, reflexology, reiki and visualisation and guided imagery. She works as a complementary nurse therapist at Beechwood Cancer Care Day Centre in Stockport, Cheshire. Barbara's special area of expertise is in combining the therapies she practises for the benefit of individual patients and carers. In addition, she is a course leader for a reflexology and cancer care course, which is a core module of the Diploma in Clinical Reflexology.

DIANE GRAY, PGCE, MAR, practises a range of therapies including aromatherapy, massage, reflexology and reiki. She is also a practitioner member of the British Flower Vibrational Essence Association. Diane has over 7 years' experience working in palliative care and she currently works as a therapist at the Macmillan Care Centre in Trafford and in the Young Oncology Unit at Christie Hospital. Diane is also qualified to teach massage, aromatherapy and baby massage.

SUE HAMPTON, CTA, has a BSc Honours degree in Biochemistry and Soil Science. She is a Certified Transactional Analyst and a Body-Centred Psychotherapist, registered with the UKCP. Sue's focus is on promoting 'super-health' with her clients by helping them to improve the effectiveness and health of their immune system. She does this holistically by using an integrated physiological, emotional and psychological approach. She also supports organisations to deal more effectively with stress and its effects.

EDWINA HODKINSON, RGN, BRCP, MAR, is the Clinical Lead for Complementary Therapy at Bury Cancer Centre, Bury, Greater Manchester, and Deputy Clinical Lead for Complementary Therapy at Christie Hospital. She has a background in general nursing, with qualifications in clinical aromatherapy and healing. She regularly runs courses and workshops on complementary therapies and cancer care.

TIMOTHY JACKSON, MSc, SRN, SCM, RNMS, Onc Cert, is Macmillan Network Nurse Director for the South East London Cancer Network. Tim completed his nurse training in 1982 and qualified as a midwife in 1984. He has worked in critical care, palliative care, pain management, radiotherapy, oncology and haemato-oncology at the Royal Marsden Hospital and University College London Hospitals (UCLH) in London. In addition, Tim has developed a complementary therapy service at UCLH.

NATALY LEBOULEUX, MA, DTM, came to England from France in 1992 and gained the Diploma in Holistic Massage in 1994. Nataly has her own massage practices in Manchester and Liverpool and has worked in palliative care since 1996. As a member of the Community Outreach Project Team based at the Neil Cliffe Cancer Care Centre, Manchester, Nataly also provides complementary therapies to patients with advanced metastatic and non-malignant diseases in their own homes in central Manchester. Nataly has studied different approaches to massage/body work and process-oriented psychology, and she teaches on massage courses.

KAREN LIVINGSTONE, MCSP, is a senior physiotherapist who has worked at the Neil Cliffe Cancer Care Centre since 1996. Many of the patients with whom Karen works have breast cancer and need help with problems that can occur post surgery. Karen is also qualified as a lymphoedema key worker, she manages the fatigue management service, and teaches healthcare professionals and students about fatigue management and symptom control.

ANITA MEHREZ, SRN, MAR, MCAR, was a sister on a neurosciences unit before entering into complementary therapies in 1999. She is a qualified aromatherapist and reflexologist and has a private practice in Manchester. Anita works at the Neil Cliffe Cancer Care Centre, Manchester, as an aromatherapist in the Symptom Control Clinic. She also provides complementary therapies to patients with advanced metastatic and non-malignant diseases in their own homes in Central Manchester as a member of the Community Outreach Project Team.

JUNE ROSEN, MCSP, originally trained as a physiotherapist and has worked in mental health, specialising in eating disorders, substance misuse, anxiety and depression. She qualified as an aromatherapist in 1995 and she currently works as a Deputy Clinical Lead for Complementary Therapy at Christie Hospital, Manchester. June's work involves providing complementary therapy mainly to patients with leukaemia and spinal cord compression.

JACQUI STRINGER, PhD, BSc, RGN, TIDHA, is Clinical Lead/Aromatherapist at Christie Hospital NHS Trust, Manchester. Jacqui's career focus has always been the care of patients with haematological or oncological conditions. Her PhD, which she completed in 2005, explored the influence of massage and aromatherapy on the stress levels of patients undergoing high-dose chemotherapy while being nursed in isolation. In 2003, Jacqui was awarded a Winston Churchill Memorial Trust Travelling Fellowship which allowed her to develop her work through visiting the USA.

PAOLA SYLT, BSc (Hons) in TCM (Acupuncture), was an Honorary Research Assistant for the Chair Massage for Carers Project at Christie Hospital, Manchester, and is currently Research Acupuncturist with Manchester University for an acupuncture/acupressure for post-cancer treatment fatigue study. Paola has a degree in traditional Chinese medicine and acupuncture from the University of Salford. She runs busy acupuncture clinics in Hartford and Lymm in Cheshire, with particular focus on acupuncture for infertility and chronic illness.

MARIANNE TAVARES, MSc, RGN, NDN, Cert Supervision, worked as a nurse for 20 years prior to specialising in complementary therapies at St Gemma's Hospice, Leeds. She is the author of the 'National Guidelines for the Use of Complementary Therapies in Supportive and Palliative Care', and the 'Guide for Writing Policies and Procedures for Complementary Therapies'. Marianne currently chairs the National Association of Complementary Therapists in Hospice and Palliative Care, and teaches on a course for complementary therapy co-ordinators.

CHERYL WHITE, Grad Dip Phys, MCSP, SRP, is a Senior Macmillan Lymphoedema Specialist Physiotherapist at Christie Hospital, Manchester and treats patients with lymphoedema secondary to cancer. She is trained in the Casley-Smith method and provides manual lymphatic drainage and multi-layer lymphoedema bandaging. Cheryl is an executive committee member of the British Lymphology Society and its newsletter advisor. She also teaches on courses on lymphoedema and its management.

Foreword

As health care practitioners, we all benefit from resources that help us to do our job better. However, it is not often that one comes across a book that combines knowledge with current research and shows us how to apply this in a caring and compassionate manner within the clinical setting. In this respect, you are holding a progressive and invaluable text written by some of the foremost practitioners in this field today.

The issues and challenges experienced by therapists working with people affected by cancer today demand a wide range of skills in clinical expertise. It also involves being aware of the need for continuing physical and emotional support of patients, their families and environment and of the therapist.

Rather than attempting to create a 'model' of health or illness management, we now recognise that our lives change markedly depending upon internal and external influences. Health and illness management is a dynamic, fluid entity extending way beyond any form of therapy. It is also contingent upon the context in which we live our lives and when ill, the treatment we receive. However we also know that the *way* in which a therapy is given forms an essential component of the healing process.

Expanding the continuum of care we offer people should quite rightly take lifestyle and relationships into account - these are the factors that provide true quality of life and help to smooth the rocky passage through illness management. This book offers an exciting perspective on the use of bodywork for people living with cancer. As such it is invaluable. It takes us another step towards developing aspects of the healing spectrum.

Peter Mackereth and Ann Carter have cleverly brought together a range of experts in order to unite touch therapies such as massage and bodywork with orthodox forms of oncology management. The result is a unique text that expands the options of care we can offer people as well as supporting and nurturing family and friends as well as therapists.

As clinical practitioners, we have all encountered situations where nothing seems to work; in the past, emphasis upon physical symptoms would have excluded ways of helping people to manage their situation. Today, we know that there is always something that can be done. We know that effective collaboration and support makes us better practitioners and better people. Team work, supervision and mentoring help us to grow and to learn. These issues also help us to reflect and gain greater insight and perspective into ourselves and how we live our lives.

The importance of collaborative, developmental and reflective support is eloquently raised in this book . It cannot be over-estimated in helping us to grow and to prevent, as Lyckholm (2001) commented, being overwhelmed by the challenges and loss that can occur when working in cancer care.

I am delighted to have been asked to write a forward for this book and I have no doubt that what you read here will inform, clarify, challenge and inspire your current practice. By reading this book you will develop your clinical skills. It will also refine the essential components of reflective practice that will guide your work and support you on your journey as you learn about massage and bodywork.

Denise Rankin-Box, Macclesfield, 2006

REFERENCE

Lyckholm L. (2001) Dealing with stress, burnout, and grief in the practice of oncology. The Lancet Oncology 2(12):750–755

Foreword

'Healing is brought about not just by medicine. It's not just treatment which cures you, but all that encompasses the human touch'

In March 1994, a lump appeared on the left side of my neck. Little did I know that I also had tumours inside my chest and in my armpit, I had been struck down with Hodgkin's disease, which is cancer of the lymph glands, I was 30 years old. Nothing I had already been through, or been taught or heard from other people, prepared me for what I was about to go through in the next 12 years. It was more difficult and painful than I had ever imagined.

'I need to know that this body is my body. And I need to know everything that is happening to my body. But most of all I need to know that you know that within my body there is me.'

Suddenly my body was out of control, my life was out of control, I felt out of control. My body no longer felt my own, attacked and threatened by this dreaded cancer, and then in the attempt to rid me and my body of this life threatening disease the onslaught of needles, scalpels, biopsies, toxic drugs, hospitals, new people, new routines, new information, trying to find a way to treat the cancer, trying to find a way through, trying to stay alive.

'What everybody has to understand is that physical illness needs emotional tendering as well as conventional treatment'

As an artist it was quite natural for me to want to express what I was experiencing through my painting, so whilst in isolation undergoing high dose chemotherapy and a peripheral stem cell (bone marrow) transplant, I started to paint the pictures that became the book 'The Emotional Cancer Journey'. Cancer is not just a medical condition but evokes an emotional response, the fear, the despair, the pain and loss, the hopes and dreams, the love and relationships, the bearable and unbearable. Cancer has brought both a terrifying reality into my life, underlied by the possibility that I might die and I have nearly died, but this facing of my shadow, my illness and death has also brought an invaluable perspective and enriching aspect to my life that I never thought possible.

What I had not realized before my illness was that there was more to cancer treatment than medicine, and that there was more ways to support care and address what was happening than tea and sympathy. I have been so lucky in the love and care that I have been given, not just by my friends and family, and the doctors, nurses and other healthcare workers but also the complementary therapists. This was a completely new world to me. Shiatsu and other body massage, reflexology, aromatherapy, acupuncture, reike healing, hypnotherapy, homeopathy and counselling. This was a different type of touch and touching. Amazing.

Fiona, one of my house mates had been diagnosed with breast cancer two years before my own diagnosis of Hodgkin's disease. She had managed to get her GP to refer her to The Royal London Homeopathic Hospital to have complementary treatment alongside the conventional medicine. I decided to do the same. There I was offered and had my first shiatsu massage. It was superb and became a regular treatment.

A year later, when I was admitted to University College Hospital in London on the haematology ward, to my amazement me and my partner were offered reflexology to help calm and nurture us. I have never looked back. This was a new world indeed. One of the first procedures that I needed was to have a Hickman line inserted into my chest, to allow the gamut of drugs, blood tests and bone marrow transplant to begin. Incredibly, an hour before being sent down to theatre for the general anaesthetic and operation again came Julia to give me reflexology. As part of this new integration, she had a schedule of operations and automatically came to see the patients beforehand to offer this service. I felt completely nurtured and it certainly helped my fear and preparation for this awful but necessary procedure.

I couldn't believe how integrated this had become in an NHS ward, just fantastic. But this was just the tip of the iceberg, not just in terms of something nice and soothing but actually addressing pain, fear, nausea, asthma, all sorts of cancer symptoms, treatment side effects and emotional issues. It has become integral and integrated to my cancer treatment and care as well as my emotional and physical welfare. This 'touch', the hands of the therapists alongside those of my doctors and nurses, and the hugs and kisses of my personal friends and carers, have 'cradled' me through the nekia, my dark nights of my cancer illness, just as my painting, 'The Cradle of the World' that illustrates the cover of this book, depicts.

Peter, Ann and their colleagues have put together this wonderful informative book for therapists. They have included case studies adapted from real life. The experience of living with cancer and its treatment is hard to describe in words. Sometimes images can help to convey feelings, fears for others to have a glimpse of the impact of cancer and its treatment. We can all learn so much from patients and therapists as they try to find the resources to cope and fight with every unimaginable situation. Complementary therapies, such as shiatsu, reflexology and aromatherapy have always helped lift my spirits. Therapists can contribute to the love that many nurses, doctors, counsellors, and even hospital cleaners, give every day to patients like me, and I am eternally grateful to all those who have contributed to my physical, medical, emotional and spiritual healing as a response to the biggest challenge in my life, my cancer.

Michele Petrone
Director of MAP Foundation, June 2006

For more information about the MAP Foundation

Website: www.mapfoundation.org
Email: info@mapfoundation.org
Registered Charity No. 1093684

REFERENCE

Petrone MA (2003) The Emotional Cancer Journey
Available from the MAP Foundation

Acknowledgements

The Editors would like to thank all the contributors who have worked tirelessly to bring this work to fruition, especially in the light of all the other personal and professional demands and challenges in their lives. Special thanks to all the patients, carers and staff, whose (anonymous) case scenarios have served to illuminate elements of the text.

Peter would like to particularly thank Stephen McGinn for his unstinting support and ability to know just when to offer an espresso coffee or a camomile tea. Peter is also extremely grateful to his colleagues, and patients and carers at Christie NHS Trust, Manchester for their help and inspiration. He also thanks Michael Smith and Jo Robinson for their encouragement and support.

Ann would like to thank the team of key workers and health professionals at the Neil Cliffe Cancer Care Centre site, St Ann's Hospice, Manchester, for their ongoing support and listening ears when they were most required. She also thanks Sandra Day whose inspiration and commitment to the use of complementary therapies in cancer care provided a foundation for many of the initiatives covered in the book.

Peter and Ann would particularly like to thank Anne Cawthorn, Gwynneth Campbell, Paula Maycock, Angela Clarke, Sally Olsberg, Clive O'Hara, Liz Tipping, Denise Rankin-Box, Caroline Hoffman, Chris Johns, Tiffany Field and Maria Hernandez-Reif, who in their way have all influenced and shaped the development of this text.

Ann and Peter would like to dedicate this book to their fathers, who both challenged and valued their work.

Introduction

The book is aimed primarily at qualified massage and bodywork therapists, in the UK and internationally, who want to expand their knowledge and skills. The number of therapists has dramatically increased since the mid 1990s, and educational establishments are also becoming more discerning about the use of the available literature. Students attending university degree and college diploma programmes are also driving the demand for evidence-based and academic texts. Additionally, teachers also want published work that is referenced and recommends further useful reading and resources. No longer is there one simple text that meets the academic and practical application of a therapy. It is now commonplace to find massage therapists who are reflexologists, and also aromatherapists. This book has brought together several approaches to bodywork with a focus on an important area of practice – palliative and supportive cancer care.

In the past, using massage and other bodywork therapies with people who have cancer has been approached with some reservations. Recent research and clinical reviews of the evidence is now supportive of touch therapies. We would like to emphasise that therapists must be able to skilfully adapt treatments for individuals, and be mindful of working collaboratively with the multidisciplinary teams. An important aspect of this text is that we have broadened the adaptations and value of massage and bodywork beyond the work with patients to include a 'bigger picture' so issues relating to the context in which therapeutic intervention take place are also covered.

This unique book will also be of value to students, teachers and postgraduates who are looking to work safely, competently, and with compassion in the field of cancer care. There are many healthcare professionals, such as nurses, physiotherapists and occupational therapists, who have trained in massage or bodywork, and who want to study further, so that their skills can be developed and integrated in clinical practice. This text will also be useful to co-ordinators of complementary therapy services, researchers, and user groups representing cancer patients. The book is also intended as a resource for clinical nurse specialists and other health professionals who provide information to patients and colleagues.

The book has been divided into two sections. The first deals with key themes which include theoretical perspectives on cancer and its treatments, a review of the research evidence for massage and bodywork, integration issues, chapters on psychological aspects of the work and the therapist in the role of teacher. All these themes are explored and discussed, utilising the available literature, analysis of models and concepts, and are related specifically to cancer care. The second section focuses on the different and most common modalities of massage and bodywork, and includes chair massage, reflexology, shiatsu and aromatherapy and how they are being adapted in practice. The authors review the therapies and how they can be adapted to a context. Concerns and challenges to the application of these approaches are also discussed.

This text takes the novice and the more experienced practitioner on a journey of examination, critical review and debate prior to making recommendations for best practice. Many of the ideas in this new book have evolved from the process and challenges of adapting practice in hospice care, as well as using the therapies in acute cancer care settings within the National Health Service. The project to write the book has also been influenced by growing public and patient interest in complementary therapy. There is an expectation that professional therapists will utilise contemporary information to support their practice, so that they can be reassured of person centred, effective, and importantly, safe service. It is important to state that any recommendations made by an author(s) are to be carefully considered by the reader and they are not a prescription to be followed without training, supervision and support. It beholds the accountable and responsible therapist to only consider an action, or inaction, in line with their codes of professional practice, where there is appropriate support of the employer/manager/supervisor and the informed consent of the client/patient. If in doubt, it is always recommended that the therapist should not proceed, and should seek advice and support. It behoves the profession to become one of critical and reflective practitioners, and to acknowledge the value of research and enquiry in this process.

To enhance the development of professional complementary therapy practice in cancer care, the Editors were concerned to communicate and disseminate their understanding and appraisal of the therapies at this time, in order to encourage objective debate. This book therefore has a strong focus on adapting practice, which emphasises key professional issues such as informed assessment of patients, reflective and supervised practice, accountability, evidence base and health and safety issues. The contributors are all involved in a variety of professional activities related to complementary therapies including practice, research, teaching and publication. Many are also qualified health professionals and include physiotherapists, nurses and psychotherapists. They are respected colleagues and fellow learners in the art and science of massage and bodywork, and as editors we would like to extend our grateful thanks to them all for their professionalism, commitment and willingness to share their expertise and experience with others.

In selecting this book for your development and studies, we feel that you are entering into a journey of exploration and discovery. We hope it will inspire you to continue learning so that you become even more creative through adapting your massage and bodywork skills. We also want the contents to support you in attaining your personal and professional potential; we are all part of a worldwide movement to acquire the necessary evidence and experience to enable true integration of complementary therapies into a variety of healthcare systems.

Ann Carter and Peter Mackereth,
2006

Key themes

Section contents

INTRODUCTION

This book, which explores the adaptations of massage and bodywork in cancer care, has been divided into two sections. The first part consists of seven chapters; each is a critical review of contemporary themes specific to this area of clinical practice. The authors have diverse backgrounds but all have skills in teaching, therapeutic/clinical work in cancer care, as well as involvement in the supervision of therapists. It is important for the reader, who may go through the chapters individually, to be aware that both sections of the book are linked. Section 2 examines the innovations in the application of the therapy in detail. There is also cross-referencing between chapters to avoid duplication of important issues and concerns.

All chapters have a short abstract and keywords. Case studies are integrated within the text to illuminate both the rationale for adaptation and the individualised nature of the work. Each chapter also includes supportive references, a list of further reading and useful addresses and contacts.

Chapter 1, Cancer and its treatment by Tim Jackson, provides an introduction to the nature of cancer and its treatments. It includes a description of the incidence of common cancers and possible causes. The signs and symptoms of cancer are listed and medical treatments are described. In Chapter 2, Integrative practice by Marianne Tavares, the integration of massage and bodywork in a hospice environment is explored. The author is an experienced coordinator, supervisor and therapist. Marianne examines the concept of integration and how teams can work, responding effectively to the needs of patients in a way which is individual, sensitive, respectful and seamless. Chapter 3, Evaluating the evidence by Jacqui Stringer and Peter Mackereth, examines the evidence in massage and bodywork, and gives examples of recently published research work. Importantly, the focus of the chapter is an exploration of key issues that arise when considering conducting research work with people affected by cancer.

In Chapter 4, Professional and potent practice by Peter Mackereth and Ann Carter, the discussion is centred on the characteristics of a profession and model of practice. Included in the content are strategies to support and encourage reflective practice, such as continuing education activities and clinical supervision. The main focus of Chapter 5, Working with the denied body by Anne Cawthorn, is the utilisation of a therapeutic model to integrate complementary and alternative medicine therapies into cancer care in a way that will safely facilitate the patient's adjustment. This is explored through the use of case studies from the author's experience as a psychotherapist. Chapter 6, Body psychotherapy in cancer care by Sue Hampton, describes body psychotherapy and its links with psychoneuroimmunology, and three different approaches to psychotherapy, and provides an outline of the methods used. The tasks of both the therapist and the patient are included.

Lastly, in Chapter 7, Therapist as teacher by Peter Mackereth, Jacqui Stringer and Diane Gray, the authors examine how, when and why professional therapists need to develop their skills in teaching and supporting parents and partners to provide massage interventions in cancer care settings. Case studies are utilised to illuminate the safe and therapeutic practice of enabling parents and partners to provide safe and therapeutic massage.

1

Cancer and its treatments

Timothy Jackson

Abstract

The chapter provides an introduction to the nature of cancer and its treatments. It includes a description of the incidence of common cancers and possible causes. The signs and symptoms of cancer are listed and medical treatments are described. The chapter is an overview and not a definitive text. The recommendations at the end of the chapter are to encourage therapists to maintain and develop their knowledge and effective multidisciplinary working.

KEYWORDS

cancer, causes, incidence, surgery, chemotherapy, radiotherapy, palliative and supportive care

THE NATURE OF CANCER

Cancer is the name given to a large group of diseases (just over 200) having common characteristics (Corner & Bailey 2001). A dictionary definition of 'cancer' has been given as: 'a class of *diseases* characterized by uncontrolled *cell* division and the ability of these cells to invade other *tissues*, either by direct growth into adjacent tissue (*invasion*) or by migration of cells to distant sites (*metastasis*)' (Hirsch et al 2002). The organs and tissues of the body are made up of tiny building blocks called cells. Cells in different parts of the body may look and work differently but most reproduce in the same way. Cells are constantly becoming old and dying, and new cells are produced to replace them. Normally the division and growth of cells is orderly and controlled but if this process gets out of control for some reason the cells will continue to divide and develop to form a tumour. Tumours can either be benign (do not spread) or malignant (spread or metastasise). Cancers can be broadly grouped into different types, depending on which tissues they come from (Box 1.1).

Box 1.1
Cancers and tissue groups

- **Carcinomas** form from cells that cover internal and external body surfaces. The most frequently occurring cancers in this group are breast, lung and colon.
- **Leukaemias** are a group of cancers which result in immature blood cells growing in the bone marrow and then they tend to accumulate in large numbers in the bloodstream.
- **Lymphomas** are cancers of the immune system arising in the lymphatic nodes and tissues.
- **Sarcomas** arise from cells found in the body's supporting tissues, such as bone, fat, connective tissue, cartilage and muscle.
- **Adenomas** are cancers that arise from glandular tissue, such as the pituitary, the thyroid and the adrenal glands. They are mostly benign.

Source: Cancer Research UK (2005).

Box 1.2
Terms used as prefixes

- Adeno = gland
- Chondro = cartilage
- Erythro = red blood cell
- Haemangio = blood vessel
- Hepato = liver
- Lipo = fat
- Lympho = white blood cell
- Melano = pigment cell
- Myelo = bone marrow
- Myo = muscle
- Osteo = bone

Source: Cancer Research UK (2005).

Terms that are used as prefixes describe the type of cell from which the cancer originated, for example an osteosarcoma is a cancer of the bone (see Box 1.2).

Some of the commonest solid cancers are breast, lung, colorectal, gynaecological and prostate cancers. Rare cancers include, for example, sarcomas, leukaemias and lymphomas. In Box 1.3 the 10 commonest cancers are listed by sex.

Box 1.3
The 10 commonest cancers in UK by sex*

Females	Males
Breast – 30%	Prostate – 20%
Colorectal (large bowel) – 12%	Lung – 17%
Lung – 11%	Colorectal (large bowel) – 14%
Ovary – 5%	Bladder – 6%
Uterus – 4%	Stomach – 5%
Stomach – 3%	Head and neck – 4%
Melanoma – 3%	Non-Hodgkin's lymphoma – 3%
Non-Hodgkin's lymphoma – 3%	Oesophagus – 3%
Pancreas – 3%	Leukaemia – 3%
Bladder – 2%	Kidney – 3%
Other – 24%	Other – 21%

Source: Cancer Research UK (2005). *Data 2000.

CAUSES AND PROGNOSIS

The aetiology of cancer is not yet fully understood, but it is thought to be caused by a combination of factors. Acknowledged factors include the use/exposure of tobacco (including passive inhalation), alcohol and drugs. Exposure to radiation (ionising and solar), genetic predisposition, contact with viruses and/or parasites, and deficiencies of the immune system. In addition, dietary factors, occupational hazards and environmental pollution have also been implicated (Corner & Bailey 2001). Some of these factors have been useful in social policies, and recommended lifestyle changes to prevent cancer include, for example, smoking cessation, healthy diet (increasing intake of fruits and vegetables and decreasing red meat consumption) and exercise to improve wellbeing (Sorensen et al 2003).

The early detection of cancer is important to ensure early treatment and improved survival. Patients may present to a therapist in private practice with possible symptoms of cancer. It is helpful if the therapist is able to encourage the patient to seek medical advice (Box 1.4).

After initial diagnosis, the term 'staging' is used to describe whether the cancer is localised, if there is nodal involvement and/or if there is metastatic spread; this can be a useful prognostic guide. Besides staging, variables such as sex or age can also be important in the progress of certain cancers. For example, children, teenagers and young adults generally present with rarer and more aggressive cancers, which may be responsive to curative high-dose therapies. In older people, some cancers may be controlled or held in remission

---

Box 1.4
Examples of signs and symptoms requiring investigation for cancer

- A new or unusual lump anywhere on the body.
- A mole which changes in shape, size or colour.
- A sore that will not heal (including in the mouth).
- A persistent problem, such as persistent coughing or hoarseness.
- A change in bowel or urinary habits.
- Any abnormal bleeding, e.g. blood in the stool or urine.
- Unexplained weight loss.

Source: Europe Against Cancer (1995).

---

with ongoing treatment modalities. For example, in men prostate cancer can be managed by endocrine treatments, with response rates of 40–80%. While not achieving a cure, it can help to contain disease progression in some individuals for a number of years (Fenlon 2001).

DIAGNOSTICS

Cancer can be diagnosed in several ways, for example following physical examination by an experienced clinician or after blood tests, such as a full blood count for leukaemia. Tests include radiological examinations (radiographs and mammography), biopsy of the tumour using endoscopy or surgery. More sophisticated diagnostic technologies such as computed tomography, magnetic resonance imaging (MRI) and positron emission tomography (PET) may also be required.

OVERVIEW OF MEDICAL TREATMENTS

Surgery

Some surgery can be diagnostic and includes biopsies and endoscopies. Definitive surgery aims to remove as much of the tumour as possible, along with a clear margin of healthy tissue that surrounds it, the purpose being to achieve a cure. Nearby lymph nodes are often removed to check for any spread of the cancer. Surgical treatments can be so extensive that removal of a tumour may require amputation of a limb or pelvic clearance of a number of organs. This has enormous implications for recovery, rehabilitation and body image. Palliative surgery is sometimes carried out to relieve symptoms of advanced cancer. It may also be necessary to insert medical devices, such as feeding tubes and stents (a rigid tube that maintains an opening in a body canal, such as the oesophagus). 'Debulking' is sometimes necessary to remove as much of the tumour as possible prior to chemotherapy or radiotherapy treatments. This process is for palliation, where the intention is to improve a patient's quality of life for as long as possible. The indications for surgery can also be prophylactic, that is, for people who have an increased genetic risk, e.g. where a woman has the breast cancer gene. In addition, some patients may also require reconstructive surgery, for example, following mastectomy.

Chemotherapy

Cytotoxic chemotherapy is the term given to drugs which kill cancer cells. Cytotoxic chemotherapy prevents the cancerous cells from developing and multiplying. Different chemotherapies are administered to prevent cell division and replication during the different stages of cell division. The aim is to maximise cell kill – this is commonly known as the 'cell kill hypothesis (Figure 1.1).

Cycles of different types of chemotherapy are given to maximise cell kill and minimise unwanted side effects. The treatment is given at regular intervals to allow recovery and at the same time prevent or minimise tumour growth. Over a period of time the tumour can be completely destroyed. Side effects are divided into short, medium and long term (Box 1.5) and vary depending on the type and dosage of chemotherapy. Cytotoxic chemotherapy affects non-cancer cells, especially those that divide rapidly, i.e. hair, mucosa and the immune system.

The side effects of chemotherapy are numerous and complex, for example neutropenia (low white cell count) leaves a patient particularly susceptible to infection. Opportunistic infections, which can present in people with

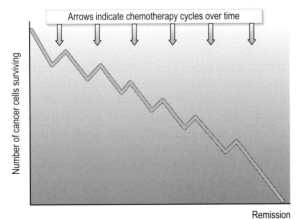

Figure 1.1   The cancer cell kill hypothesis with chemotherapy.

Box 1.5
Side effects of chemotherapy

Monitoring for prompt recognition for signs and symptoms of side effects and immediate treatment and care is paramount in oncology patients. The side effects include:

- **Immediate:** anaphylaxis, nausea, vomiting, chemical cystitis, flushing.
- **Short and medium term:** diarrhoea, constipation, dry mouth, loss of appetite, anorexia, peripheral neuropathy, menopause, loss of sleep, altered body image.
- **Long term:** hair loss, altered body image, loss of function, infertility, anaemia, neutropenia, thrombocytopenia (haemorrhage) or pancytopenia, insomnolence, cardiac/renal/hepatic impairment, premature menopause, psychological and sociological effects.
- **Rare side effects:** kidney damage, liver damage, heart failure including cardiac conduction and cardiomyopathy, peripheral neuropathy (tingling in the hands and feet), damage to the bladder lining, tinnitus.

Dougherty & Bailey (2001), Stein (2003).

functioning immune systems, severely compromise the neutropenic patient. These include bacterial infections, viral infections such as herpes zoster or shingles, or fungal infections such as aspergillus. Infection may be detected on physical examination of the skin, mouth, and intravenous sites. It can be difficult to assess in patients with low white blood cell counts as there may be no signs of inflammation. In the neutropenic patient who has a systemic infection, there may only be evidence of a raised temperature. A temperature of 38°C or above requires immediate treatment with powerful intravenous antibiotics. If left untreated, septic shock may develop and death may occur within a few hours or days. Regular analysis of the urine for blood or protein can indicate if there is an infection and further microscopic testing of the blood may be required. Patient information is key to recognising and alerting health professionals to side effects which require specialist treatment and care. It is important also to provide information to patients to enable them to understand their disease and its treatment, so that they can make choices about their care. The side effects caused by chemotherapy may require additional supportive care and/or further medication. Examples of conventional treatments to manage side effects are given in Box 1.6.

Hormones

Hormonal therapy can play a part in the management of cancer and its symptoms. It can be given to treat and/or control certain cancers such as breast

> **Box 1.6**
> **Examples of conventional management for side effects of chemotherapy**
>
> - Anti-emetics for nausea and vomiting.
> - Analgesia for pain, plus other drugs known as co-analgesics (e.g. steroids can help to reduce swelling and inflammation, which in turn reduces pain).
> - Intravenous fluids for dehydration (e.g. due to diarrhoea or nausea and vomiting), plus additional minerals such as potassium or calcium for electrolyte disturbances.
> - Aperients or laxatives for constipation.
> - Blood product transfusion such as packed red cells for anaemia or platelets to prevent or stop bleeding.
> - Antibiotics, antiviral drugs, antifungal drug therapy for infections.
>
> Edwards (2003).

or prostate cancers. The therapy leads to a fall in the levels of certain hormones that would otherwise cause increased tumour size and activity. Tumours can also be complicated by local inflammation and oedema, which can obstruct nerve pathways and cause pain and/or alteration in sensation.

Steroids

Steroids, such as synthetic glucocorticoids, have potent anti-inflammatory actions that can reduce oedema around the tumour (Guerrero 1998). Steroids given in high doses suppress the immune system and therefore when combined with high dose chemotherapy are used in the treatment of acute leukaemias. These therapies do have side effects; for example, steroids can increase blood sugar, reduce immunity, alter deposition of fat, and affect mood and appetite. Patients need to be provided with information about these effects and any alteration must be monitored and supervised by the patient's physician.

Radiotherapy

Radiotherapy is an intervention that uses ionising radiation, the goal being to destroy or inactivate cancer cells while preserving the integrity of the normal tissues surrounding the tumour (Dunne-Daly 1999). A machine called a linear accelerator, which looks like a large x-ray machine, delivers radiotherapy. The treatment is measured in units called fractions that usually takes several minutes to complete. Treatment planning takes into account a number of factors including the cancer site(s), radiotherapy sensitivity and staging. The total dose can be divided over weeks. Patients must be placed in the exact position for the treatment with the area(s) marked. Immobilisation and positioning devices, such as masks, casts and arm boards, are sometimes necessary to ensure stabilisation and accuracy (Faithfull 2001).

Sometimes brachytherapy is given; this involves radioactive sources positioned within a body cavity, or tissue close to the tumour. The tumour then receives a higher dose, with less radiation affecting the surrounding healthy tissue. These sealed sources can be left in position for a few minutes or a few hours. This treatment is used for certain cancers such as tongue, breast, uterine and cervical cancers (Dunn-Daly 1999, Faithfull 2001).

Radioactive liquids (unsealed source therapy) are given as an injection or a drink and target a particular type of tissue, e.g. radioactive iodine for thyroid cancer, radioactive strontium for prostate cancer which has spread to the bones, and radioactive phosphorous for certain malignant blood disorders. Caesium-125 is a radioactive element that is put into an applicator and then inserted into the cervix and vagina. This is known as caesium insertion and patients undergo this procedure under a general anaesthetic. Some patients will have caesium insertion and are connected to a Selectron machine. This loads the radioactive material into the applicator once the patient has returned from theatre. Patients are nursed in isolation, following strict radiation protection guidelines and policies (Dunn-Daly 1999). Treatment lasts for 12–48 hours and the patient is observed on closed circuit television. Opening the door to the room switches off the machine so any undue interruptions will prolong the length of time in isolation, which can be distressing for the patient.

SIDE EFFECTS OF RADIOTHERAPY

Patients receiving radiotherapy may experience two common side effects: skin reactions and fatigue. Skin reactions are site specific, and the skin in the treatment field may become reddened and sore. Patients are advised to wear loose clothing and use non-scented toiletries. If the skin reaction is severe, the treatment may have to be temporarily suspended. Fatigue is recognised as a common occurrence with radiotherapy, and usually begins during treatment and can persist for days and even weeks (Ahlberg et al 2005, Molassiotis & Chan 2004). The causes of fatigue are not fully understood, but may be due to the accumulation of metabolites of cell destruction and the need for resources for tissue repair (Faithfull 2001).

ROLE OF SUPPORTIVE AND PALLIATIVE CARE

Cancer is a complex illness with regard to its aetiology, spread and the application of medical treatments. Supportive care has been defined as that which 'helps the patient and his/her family to cope with cancer and treatment of it – from pre-diagnosis, through the process of diagnosis and treatment, to cure, continuing illness or death and into bereavement. It helps the patient to maximize the benefits of treatment and to live as well as possible with the effects of the disease. It is given equal priority alongside diagnosis and treatment' (NICE 2004). The National Council for Hospice Supportive and Palliative Care Services in the National Institute for Health and Clinical Excellence (NICE) guidance (2004) has identified multidisciplinary approaches to supportive care (Box 1.7).

Box 1.7
Supportive care

Multidisciplinary approaches can be offered at any stage of the illness. These include:

- User involvement – self-help and support
- Information giving
- Psychological support
- Symptom control
- Social support
- Rehabilitation
- Complementary therapies
- Spiritual support
- Palliative care
- End-of-life and bereavement care

NICE (2004).

Palliative care

Palliative is derived from 'pallium', an adjective meaning 'cloaked' or 'concealed' and a verb meaning 'to cloak', 'to clothe', or 'to shelter' (Webster's Medical Dictionary 2003). It is a term often used where disease is advanced, although this approach to care is argued as useful throughout the cancer journey (Pennell & Corner 2001). Palliative care has been defined by NICE (2004) as 'the active holistic care of patients with advanced, progressive illness' (p. 20). Its aim is to maximise quality of life for patient and carers and includes the management of pain and other symptoms alongside provision of other forms of support of an emotional, psychological or spiritual nature. Palliative care can also be offered at an earlier stage of illness if appropriate, in conjunction with other treatments. This may be a cause of concern to some patients and their families as palliation is often associated with advanced disease and for patients who are dying. Some of the aims of palliative care are listed in Box 1.8.

> ## Box 1.8
> ### Aims of palliative care
>
> - Provide relief from pain and other distressing symptoms.
> - Integrate the psychological and spiritual aspects of patient care.
> - Offer a support system to help patients to live as actively as possible until death.
> - To help the family to cope during the patient's illness and in their own bereavement.
> - To be applied early in the course of illness in conjunction with other therapies intended to prolong life (such as chemotherapy or radiation therapy), including investigations to better understand and manage distressing clinical side effects.
>
> NICE (2004, p. 20).

There may be overlap between supportive and palliative care, such as where there are complex and unresolved issues. These may include the management of distressing symptoms, as well as difficult psychosocial concerns. The latter may encompass end-of-life and bereavement issues. It is important to acknowledge that some patients may also live with cancer for some years, accessing hospital and hospice care for assessment and palliative care on an intermittent basis. Living longer and (hopefully) better with enduring cancers requires services to accommodate patients who are 'surviving' yet acutely aware of their own mortality. Increasingly patients and their carers are being encouraged to take a greater role in managing and evaluating services and treatments (NICE 2004).

SUMMARY

Complementary therapists are likely to be working very closely with patients living with cancer. This overview of cancer and its treatments provides information about the cancer journey from a conventional treatment perspective. Readers are encouraged to widen their knowledge by reading the literature and undertaking further training (see Useful Reading below). The recommendations listed in Box 1.9 are to guide therapists in their understanding of the complexities of cancer and its treatment.

ACKNOWLEDGEMENT

Angela Clark, Team Leader, St Ann's Hospice, the Neil Cliffe Cancer Care Centre, Manchester.

Box 1.9
Recommendations

- Massage therapists should be fully conversant with cancer treatments and their potential side effects in order to work within the boundaries of safe practice.
- Organisations and institutions should ensure that there are facilities for therapists to learn about medical treatments.
- Therapists also need to appreciate the physical, emotional and spiritual issues involved in integrated cancer care, which includes the processes and effects of diagnosis and treatment.
- It is essential that massage therapists keep up to date with new developments in cancer treatments to maintain their knowledge and adapt their treatments accordingly.
- It is useful for therapists to have an understanding of cancer treatments to facilitate effective communication and multidisciplinary working.
- Knowledge of conventional diagnosis and treatment also enhances a therapist's understanding of the patient's (and carer(s)) experiences and challenges of living with cancer.
- Therapists need to work in collaboration with other health professionals to improve the patient (and carer) experience.

REFERENCES

Ahlberg K, Ekman T, Gaston-Johansson F 2005 The experience of fatigue, other symptoms and global quality of life during radiotherapy for uterine cancer. International Journal of Nursing Studies 42:377–386

Cancer Research UK, Information Resource Centre. Online. Available: http://info.cancerresearchuk.org. (accessed 14 October 2005)

Corner J, Bailey C 2001 Cancer nursing: care in context. Blackwell Science Ltd, Oxford

Dougherty L, Bailey C 2001 Chemotherapy. In: Corner J, Bailey C (eds) Cancer nursing: care in context. Blackwell Science Ltd, Oxford

Dunne-Daly CF 1999 Principles of radiotherapy and radiobiology. Seminars in Oncology Nursing 15(4):250–259

Edwards SJ 2003 Prevention and treatment of adverse effects related to chemotherapy for recurrent ovarian cancer. Seminars in Oncology Nursing 19(3 Suppl 1):19–39

Europe Against Cancer 1995 European 10-Point Code. Working Party on European Code, London

Faithfull S 2001 Radiotherapy. In: Corner J, Bailey C (eds) Cancer nursing: care in context. Blackwell Science Ltd, Oxford

Fenlon D 2001 Endocrine therapies. In: Corner J, Bailey C (eds) Cancer nursing: care in context. Blackwell Science Ltd, Oxford

Guerrero D (ed) 1998 Neuro-oncology for nurses. Whurr Publications, London

Hirsch ED Jr, Kett JF, Trefil J (eds) 2002 The new dictionary of cultural literacy, 3rd edn. Houghton Mifflin Company, Boston, MA

Molassiotis A, Chan CWH 2004 Fatigue patterns in Chinese patients receiving radiotherapy. European Journal of Oncology Nursing 8:334–340

National Audit Office 2005. Tackling cancer in England. Saving more lives. NAO, London

National Institute for Clinical Excellence 2004 Improving supportive and palliative care for adults with cancer: the manual. National Institute for Clinical Excellence, London

Pennell M, Corner J 2001 Palliative care and cancer. In: Corner J, Bailey C (eds) Cancer nursing: care in context. Blackwell Science Ltd, Oxford

Sorensen G, Emmons K, Hunt MK et al 2003 Model for incorporating social context in health behaviour interventions: applications for cancer prevention for working-class, multi-ethnic populations. Preventive Medicine 37(3): 188–197

Stein KD, Denniston M, Baker F et al 2003 Validation of a Modified Rotterdam Symptom Checklist for use with cancer patients in the United States. Journal of Pain and Symptom Management 26(5):975–989

Webster's New World Medical Dictionary 2003 2nd edn. John Wiley & Sons Ltd, Chichester

FURTHER READING

National Institute for Clinical Excellence 2004 Improving supportive and palliative care for adults with cancer: the manual. National Institute for Clinical Excellence, London

Corner J, Bailey C 2001 Cancer nursing: care in context. Blackwell Science Ltd, Oxford

USEFUL ADDRESSES

Cancer BACUP
3 Bath Place
Rivington Street
London EC2A 3JR
UK

National Institute for Clinical Excellence
Website: www.nice.org.uk

Integrative practice

2

Marianne Tavares

Abstract

Significant shifts in health awareness and expectations of healthcare systems in the last 20 years have led to a more critical appraisal of healthcare provision and a demand for more information by the general public. Alongside this trend has been the rise in self-help measures, particularly complementary therapies. The value placed on complementary therapies by patients with cancer is implicit in the use of the therapies by patients, and the increasing provision by public healthcare organisations. A natural progression is to examine how these therapies can be more fully integrated into supportive and palliative care services. This chapter explores the integration of massage and bodywork in a hospice environment where there is an inpatient unit.

KEYWORDS

integration, accountability, evidence-based practice, multidisciplinary approach, skilful touch, sources of referral

INTRODUCTION

The term 'integrated care' is used in different situations to mean different things. In this chapter, 'integrated care' is understood primarily as an approach to care which incorporates the use of complementary therapies alongside conventional healthcare approaches. Surveys have shown that it is the 'touch' therapies – massage, aromatherapy and reflexology – that are most widely provided in cancer care in the UK (Macmillan Cancer Relief 2002). It is important to remember that integrated care attempts to understand the person as a 'whole', an approach that encompasses body, mind and spirit within a social and cultural context. The approach involves all healthcare professionals working as a team, in partnership with the patient – paying particular attention to the person's lifestyle and the quality of their relationships (Rees & Weil 2001). The philosophy of supportive and palliative care recognises the

importance of psychological/emotional, spiritual and social needs and priorities, and an integrated approach recognises the impact that these needs may
have on symptom control (Twycross 1997).

Bodywork is a general term referring to more than 30 different types of
therapy (see Chapter 6) that involve touching a person's body in a particular
way for therapeutic purposes (Russell 1994). Massage is one form of bodywork. It has been observed that an effective massage intervention is not just
a simple 'backrub' but a specialised skill that requires training as well as affective and cognitive investment on the part of the practitioner (Ferrell-Torry &
Glick 1993).

'Supportive and palliative care' is the current terminology used in the UK
to describe what has previously been known as 'palliative care'. Palliative care
is the active holistic care of patients with advanced, progressive illness, but
many aspects of palliative care are also applicable earlier in the course of
the person's illness (National Council for Hospice and Specialist Palliative
Care Services (NCHSPCS) 2002). Supportive care refers to that care which
helps patients and their families cope with cancer and its treatment, from
pre-diagnosis through the process of diagnosis and treatment to cure, continuing illness or death and into bereavement (NCHSPCS 2002, National
Institute for Clinical Excellence (NICE) 2004).

The three main elements to be considered when integrating massage and
bodywork in supportive and palliative care are: accountability, evidence-based
practice and the multidisciplinary approach. Much has already been written
about accountability and evidence-based practice (Foundation for Integrated
Medicine (FIM) 1997, House of Lords 2000, Stone 2002, Tavares 2003). Although
this chapter will discuss these issues, the main focus will be on integration at
the level of the multidisciplinary team.

ACCOUNTABILITY

The culture of 'accountability' has been significantly strengthened in the previous decade since the publication of the government's strategy for ensuring
that quality of care becomes the driving force for the development of health
services in England (Department of Health (DoH) 1997, 1998). The framework
of clinical governance provides health service organisations with clear direc-
tives on what constitutes commitment to quality and the safeguarding of
standards (DoH 1999). Integration of massage and bodywork therapies therefore involves a commitment to quality within the current framework of clinical
governance. This involves:

- Clear lines of responsibility and accountability for the overall quality
  of the service provided.
- Availability of a comprehensive programme of quality improvement
  activities, such as:

- audit and evaluation of service
- routine application of evidence-based practice
- implementation of the recently published NICE guidance for supportive and palliative care, particularly the section on complementary therapy (NICE 2004)
- processes and standards for assuring the quality of clinical care, including effective monitoring systems
- participation in well-designed relevant research.
- Availability of policies aimed at managing risks.
- Availability of agreed procedures to identify and remedy poor performance.

In practice, this commitment to quality involves a number of 'best practice' recommendations (Box 2.1).

The recommendations, although not an exhaustive list, have been developed from a variety of sources including An Ethical Framework for Complementary and Alternative Therapists (Stone 2002); the National Guidelines for the Use of Complementary Therapies in Supportive and Palliative Care (Tavares 2003); Guidance on Cancer Services: Improving Supportive and Palliative Care for Adults with Cancer (NICE 2004); and the Guide for Writing Policies, Procedures and Protocols (Tavares 2005).

Box 2.1
Quality services: recommendations for best practice

- Appointment of therapists (paid and volunteer) who are registered and insured to practise.
- Induction and training of therapists (paid and volunteer) to work in supportive and palliative care.
- Commitment of therapists (paid and volunteer) to continuing professional development.
- Clarification of ethical standards expected of therapists (paid and volunteer).
- Supervision of therapists (paid and volunteer).
- Individual performance review or appraisal of therapists.
- Clear lines of responsibility for the management of therapists (paid and volunteer).
- Development of policies, procedures and protocols.
- Regular audit and evaluation of service.
- Provision of written information for patients and their carers.
- Commitment to developing and agreeing standards at the level of the regional cancer/supportive and palliative care network.

EVIDENCE-BASED PRACTICE

Evidence-based care has been described as the conscientious, explicit and judicious use of current best evidence in making decisions about the care of individual patients (Sackett et al 1996). This understanding of evidence-based care allows massage and bodywork therapists to integrate the best available evidence with their clinical expertise, along with the patient's choice, when deciding on the form, location, duration, intensity and frequency of massage. The best available evidence for the use of massage in supportive and palliative care (Tavares 2003) shows that massage therapy has a role in supporting patients, alongside other treatments and care in numerous situations, including:

- Stress, tension and difficulties in relaxing.
- Psychological distress, e.g. anxiety, panic, low mood/depression.
- Physical symptoms, e.g. pain, nausea, breathlessness.
- Adjustment to different/changing body image.
- Sleep disturbance.
- Side effects of chemotherapy.
- Other problems that affect quality of life and wellbeing such as fatigue, adjustment to changing self-image, feelings of 'not coping'.

In addition to the best available 'published' evidence, it is vital that local providers evaluate their massage service and disseminate results to the clinical team. Participation in quality research, audit and practice inquiry (e.g. evaluation projects, practitioner reflection, user feedback) activities further promotes credibility and integration. Alongside the use of best available evidence is clinical competence. A number of factors contribute to the development of the massage and bodywork therapist's clinical expertise. These include training, commitment and experience in:

(1) The practice of massage and bodywork in supportive and palliative care.
(2) Mentoring and supervision.
(3) Continuing professional development.
(4) Multidisciplinary teamwork.

The National Guidelines for the Use of Complementary Therapies in Supportive and Palliative Care (Tavares 2003) provide useful information on the clinical issues for which training may be required (see also Chapter 4).

MULTIDISCIPLINARY APPROACH

Integrating massage and bodywork goes beyond accountability and evidence-based practice. The starting point is when massage and bodywork achieve recognition by the multidisciplinary team as a therapy that can contribute to symptom relief, psychological/emotional and spiritual care. The delivery of integrated care demands a willingness to collaborate from both conventional and complementary therapy professionals. In turn, collaboration is helped by familiarisation, understanding, and respect for, the different and overlapping roles within the team. There are key/core roles and expertise in each profession. For example, one would not expect a social worker to assess a patient's mobility, or a massage therapist to assess a patient's ability to perform tasks involved in daily living. However, some skills are shared by many professions, for example nurses may also have massage and bodywork skills. Relaxation and reduction in anxiety are some of the results of massage; however, specific techniques used by occupational therapists, physiotherapists and some counsellors also share these desired outcomes. Despite this overlapping of skills and boundaries, the contribution of each profession is unique and brings its own perspective and approaches.

It has been said that no one profession has a monopoly in responding to patients' emotional, spiritual and practical concerns (Chartered Society of Physiotherapy (CSP) 2003, Munroe 1998, NCHSPCS 2002). For example, psychological and spiritual support is provided by all professionals at levels which differ according to role and skills (NICE 2004). It is important that staff recognise the level of support they are qualified to provide. Central to teamwork is the ability by all staff to appreciate when they have reached the boundaries of their skills and to acknowledge the expertise of other members of the team. In addition, shared beliefs and goals, an agreed philosophy of care, alongside regular meetings of the multidisciplinary team helps to build a trusting working relationship between the different professionals. The challenge for professionals is to remain focused on what helps the patient, by developing an attitude which recognises the complexities of a given patient scenario and a commitment to work with the blurring, rather than a rigid attachment to role (Ryden 2001). Placing the patients and their carer(s) at the centre of service delivery is more likely to encourage collaboration, than is rivalry or protectionism of roles and titles.

The recognition of what is essentially a synergistic and integrated approach to delivering care cannot be overstated. A synergistic and integrated approach is one which recognises that the care provided by professionals working as a team is greater than that provided by the sum of individuals working on their own. For example, massage and bodywork may help patients to feel sufficiently better in themselves to be able to choose to engage in rehabilitation activities (see Case study 2.1).

Case study 2.1

A therapist was asked to see a man who was fed up and wanted to go home. However, his wife needed him to be able to transfer from bed to chair, and vice versa, before she could manage caring for him at home. The man told the therapist that he wanted to be more independent, but she was aware that so far he had been very reluctant to engage in rehabilitation activities. While massaging

> *his legs, she encouraged him to visualise himself at home transferring from bed to wheelchair and back again. The massage and visualisation was a positive and uplifting experience for the man. Later that afternoon it was reported that he started to work on his mobility with a physiotherapist.*

Effective teamwork involves the recognition of the skills of individual practitioners, and their willingness to respond in different circumstances. Case study 2.2 shows how nursing staff learned to appreciate and use the skills and approach of an experienced massage therapist in helping an anxious and distressed patient, and felt able to ask for assistance. This potent use of touch is discussed further in Chapter 8.

Case study 2.2

A nurse stopped a therapist in the corridor, saying, 'So glad I've caught you. Can you come and help with Carey who has just arrived and is in a total panic?'. The therapist agreed and found herself sitting at the edge of the bed, supporting and gently rocking Carey, using gentle massage strokes and saying repeatedly: 'It's OK, you don't have to lie down or stay still, you're OK as you are . . . you're not alone and you're very safe'. Carey began to calm down, and eventually settled, with the help of medication.

The 'panic' described in Case study 2.2, although not obvious on admission, was the restlessness that some people experience at the end of life.

Massage and bodywork practitioners can be part of a larger team providing holistic care. Table 2.1 gives a brief overview of the key roles within the multidisciplinary team. Some of these roles, e.g. rehabilitative approaches, are still evolving (NICE 2004). The purpose of outlining the key roles and responsibilities in this chapter is to aid familiarisation, and to give information which can act as a guide for referral and review purposes. Over and above core professional roles, additional or extended roles often depend on the skills and expertise of individuals, and therapists need to be familiar with the actual team members with whom they are working.

MASSAGE AS AN EMPOWERING EXPERIENCE

The key role of the massage therapist involves the use of 'skilful touch' which is offered to the patient in the form of massage. The terms 'skilful touch', 'essential touch' and 'the art of aware communication using touch' (Juhan 1987, Smith 1990, Tavares 1998, Westland 1993) have been used to describe touch which is 'sensory education', with the practitioner as facilitator. Skilful touch is said to stimulate self-awareness, re-awaken the sense of self that is beyond the physical, and restore in the person some sense of control in a seemingly powerless situation. This touch is outside of, and additional to the

Table 2.1
Roles within the multidisciplinary team

Profession	Key role	Responsibilities
Medical team	Symptom assessment and treatment of physical and psychological/emotional needs	Holistic assessment Setting goals and making decisions about overall treatment plan Arriving at end-of-life decisions Involving multidisciplinary team
Nursing team	Caring for, monitoring and supporting the patient (and carers) over 24-hour period	Holistic assessment. Providing 24-hour care Involving multidisciplinary team
Occupational therapist	Facilitating and maximising patients' functional independence at different stages of their illness and helping them to adjust to their condition	Assessment of functional difficulties in relation to activities of daily living (including home assessments), need for aids and equipment Development of coping strategies, e.g. for fatigue, anxiety, and time management; relaxation training Discharge planning when there are functional problems
Physiotherapist	Assess and treat patients to maximise their physical functioning and help them to adjust to their condition	Assessment of mobility and need for exercises, passive movements, aids and equipment, strategies for safe handling and moving, positioning (including home assessments) Respiratory care, especially breathlessness Management of lymphoedema Discharge planning when there are mobility problems

Table 2.1 continued over

Table 2.1
Roles within the multidisciplinary team—cont'd

Profession	Key role	Responsibilities
Social worker	Assess, support and explore solutions to social and psychological health/problems of the patients and their families before and after death	Acting as patient's agent with state institutions, as needed, e.g. with legal and financial matters; assistance with living at home Psychological support and counselling Bereavement support
Spiritual care team	The provision of care which facilitates patients' search for the ultimate meaning of their life, in the context of their personal belief system. To facilitate ritual which is meaningful to the patients and their carers	To ensure the provision of spiritual care, either directly or through supporting members of the multidisciplinary team To ensure patients are able to choose when they want to talk, and whom they want to talk and share with To educate staff on indications of the need for spiritual care, and about different cultural expressions and needs To support staff
Massage and bodywork therapists	The skilful use of touch for relaxation and support, and to assist in the management of symptoms and psychological and spiritual care	To work alongside other health professionals to respond to the physical, psychological and spiritual needs of patients To recognise when skilful touch and non-verbal communication may be of help to patients To educate staff on indications of need for massage and bodywork to complement other treatments

patient's personal care needs (see Chapter 8). Patients with cancer go through 'outer and inner journeys' (Thomas 2004). It is acknowledged that patients may respond to skilful touch by entering into a deep silence during massage, which can facilitate their inner journey of healing (Mackereth 1999, Tavares 1998). Skilful touch provides the time and space for patients to respond by discovering or rediscovering inner resources, strengths and often the control to respond better to the next challenge. The process and the response can be non-verbal as the person may be unable to find words to quite describe the experience, other than feeling 'very relaxed'. Appearances often change in a positive way, which may reflect inner change. Subsequent emotions, actions and decisions similarly may indicate that the individual has 'moved on'. Importantly Miller (1983) has identified hope and self-esteem to be influential elements in alleviating powerlessness in chronic illness. The experience of receiving massage may help to boost patients' self-esteem, which can in turn promote confidence in becoming more proactive in their own care.

'Touch' is a medium through which powerful emotions can surface, and the massage therapist's role is to listen, support and contain these emotions during the session. At the end of the session, it may be appropriate to discuss a referral for counselling or to a member of the spiritual care team. However, individuals may want to continue with the massage therapist for support rather than involve another professional. While it is essential to listen and be able to respond, it is important to remember one's competencies, particularly when the contract is for massage, and not counselling. Confidentiality may be understood to be 'within the team'. Nevertheless therapists need to understand that what needs to be shared is on a 'need-to-know' basis and how to document this information. Case study 2.3 shows how a therapist's skills and understanding of the patient's belief system enabled integration of massage and spiritual care.

Case study 2.3

Bridget, whose cancer had recurred, asked specifically to see the massage therapist. Bridget did not know what she was feeling, but was aware of being 'just generally down', and could not pray. She was a woman whose faith and traditional prayers were very important to her. At some point in the massage it was noticed that her eyelids were blinking rapidly; this continued for some time. The therapist asked her gently what was happening. Bridget said that she thought her previously unknown feeling was 'fear'; after she had talked about this for a while, the therapist suggested that she to 'talk to God', in prayer. The flickering of her eyelids gradually stopped, and then after the massage, Bridget said that a vision had come to her as the parable of the storm in the sea with Jesus calming the storm. Once Bridget was aware that the feeling was fear, she knew what she needed and no longer felt so helpless and depressed. On a second visit Bridget said she felt able to pray again and also talk more with her family about her feelings.

The next example shows how massage and bodywork may have enabled a carer to make greater use of her counselling sessions (Case study 2.4). Massage may have helped to 'unlock' this carer's resistance to counselling, but another perspective is that massage may also have facilitated this carer's inner journey, and boosted her self-esteem so that she was then able to face painful issues with her counsellor.

Case study 2.4

After several sessions with Irene, an assertive and determined carer, the therapist felt that Irene needed counselling support. When this was suggested to Irene the following day, she told the therapist that she had also realised this, and had just made an appointment with the counsellor. Irene's social worker confirmed this and also told the therapist that she had not taken up a previous referral for counselling. On returning for her next massage treatment Irene reported that she had been able to share her painful issues with the counsellor and felt more able to cope and receive support.

Touch therapies such as massage and reflexology have been known to 'unlock' patients' unique stress response pattern, resulting in a verbalisation of emotions, with a potential for catharsis when practised by therapists with facilitative skills (Mackereth 1999). However, there are times when massage intervention should be used with caution, and may even be contraindicated, for example with a patient or carer whose mental/emotional health is particularly fragile, and whose behaviour and responses are unpredictable. The art and skill of massage has its own potency, facilitating the body to process information and emotions non-verbally. Massage is also perhaps one of the few occasions when patients and carers can receive care without the expectation to engage in meaningful conversation the whole time.

CHALLENGES FOR THE MASSAGE AND BODYWORK THERAPIST

For massage and bodywork therapies to be more fully integrated in supportive and palliative care, therapists need to develop additional skills through education, training and supervision. Integration requires more than just providing the therapy. In summary, therapists need to be able to:

● Modify the assessment, depending on the patient's condition, and where the treatment is provided.
● Adapt the treatment according to the patient's condition and position of comfort. Treatment may be limited to 'gentle stroking' which, when practised skilfully, can be safe and yet effective.
● Assess frequency of treatment, balancing needs, resources, the environment and safety; therapists need to be aware of 'whose needs are being met' when determining frequency of treatment.

- Communicate with patients caringly, without colluding or giving 'false hope'.
- Recognise emotional distress and be able to relate to patients who are anxious, distressed, sad, depressed, angry or withdrawn.
- Recognise when a patient does not want to/need to talk.
- Recognise that the mood and condition of patients may fluctuate and adapt support safely and sensitively.
- Teach simple massage to carers and other professionals, where possible (see Chapter 7).
- Document, evaluate and communicate with the multidisciplinary team, including any need for referral to other professions.
- Being open to reflective practice, continuing education and supervision.

SOURCES OF REFERRAL

Figure 2.1 shows typical examples of services and professionals who may make referrals to a massage and bodywork therapist. The understanding of these professionals of how massage may help varies. To promote understanding and facilitate appropriate referrals, it is useful to have referral criteria. The National Guidelines for the Use of Complementary Therapies in Supportive and Palliative Care (Tavares 2003) outline the best available evidence for the use of massage and other touch therapies.

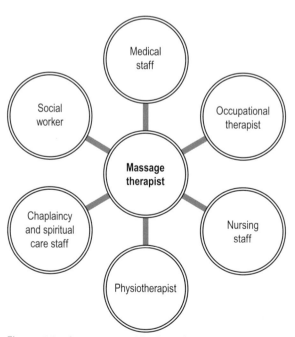

Figure 2.1   A massage and bodywork therapist can receive referrals from several sources.

Apart from referral criteria, there is a need for constant education – informal and repetitive – so that the multidisciplinary team 'remembers' the availability of massage and how it may help patients. Evaluation of the massage service from the patient's perspective and dissemination of results to the team promote understanding. Communication (formal and informal) with the nursing and medical staff, giving and receiving feedback, participation at multidisciplinary forums are useful points of promoting integration for massage services. At the organisational level, full integration is achieved when massage and bodywork therapists are employed, so that the service is not dependent on the goodwill and availability of skilled volunteer therapists. To encourage the employment of therapists, it may be helpful to obtain an agreement regarding the development of a strategy for the complementary therapy service.

SUMMARY

Integration happens at two levels – at the level of organisational management and at the level of clinical provision of services. At the organisational level accountability within the framework of clinical governance promotes credibility and support. For further integration it is useful to work towards an agreed strategy for the development of complementary therapies. At the clinical level it is important that practice is evidence based and integrated within the multidisciplinary team. Integration needs to happen in the routine of everyday care, so that massage and bodywork are no longer seen as 'something new, additional, different or special', but a profession amongst many. Integrated care is an organic and dynamic approach, and its synergistic effect enables health and social care professionals to respond as a team to the needs of patients in a way which is individual, sensitive, respectful, effective and seamless.

ACKNOWLEDGEMENTS

The author would like to thank Trish Corcoran, Advanced Nurse Practitioner, St Gemma's Hospice, Freda Magee, Vice Chair, National Association of Complementary Therapists in Hospice and Palliative Care, and Julieann Carter, Director of Nursing, St Gemma's Hospice, for their comments on the various drafts.

REFERENCES

Chartered Society of Physiotherapy 2003 The role of physiotherapy for people with cancer – CSP position statement. Chartered Society of Physiotherapy, London

Department of Health 1997 The new NHS: modern, dependable. CM 3807, The Stationery Office, London

Department of Health 1998 A first class service: quality in the new NHS. Online. Available: http://www.open.gov.uk/DOH/public/quality.htm

Department of Health 1999 Clinical governance: quality in the new NHS. NHS Executive, Department of Health, Leeds

Ferrell-Torry A, Glick O 1993 The use of therapeutic massage as a nursing intervention to modify anxiety and the perception of cancer pain. Cancer Nursing 16(2):93–101

Foundation for Integrated Medicine. Integrated healthcare – a way forward for the next five years? A discussion document. Foundation for Integrated Medicine, London

House of Lords Select Committee on Science and Technology 2000 Complementary and alternative medicine. HL Paper 123. The Stationery Office, London

Juhan D 1987 Job's body: a handbook for bodywork. Station Hill Press, New York

McKechnie AA, Wilson F, Watson N et al 1983 Anxiety states: a preliminary report on the value of connective tissue massage. Journal of Psychosomatic Research 27(2):125–129

Mackereth P 1999 An introduction to catharsis and the healing crisis in reflexology. Complementary Therapies in Nursing and Midwifery 5(3): 67–74

Macmillan Cancer Relief 2002 Directory of Complementary Therapy Services in UK Cancer Care. Macmillan Cancer Relief, London

Miller JF 1983 Coping with chronic illness. FA Davis Co, Philadelphia

Munroe B 1998 Social work in palliative care. In: Doyle D, Hanks GWC, MacDonald N (eds) Oxford Textbook of Palliative Medicine, 2nd edn. Oxford University Press, Oxford

National Council for Hospice and Specialist Palliative Care Services 2000 Raising the standard – clinical governance for voluntary hospices. National Council for Hospice and Specialist Palliative Care Services, London

National Council for Hospice and Specialist Palliative Care Services 2002 Definitions of supportive and palliative care – a consultation paper. National Council for Hospice and Specialist Palliative Care Services, London

National Council for Hospice and Specialist Palliative Care Services 2002. Turning Theory into Practice – Practical Clinical Governance for Voluntary Hospices. National Council for Hospice and Specialist Palliative Care Services, London

National Institute for Clinical Excellence 2004 Guidance on cancer services: improving supportive and palliative care for adults with cancer. National Institute for Clinical Excellence, London

Rees L, Weil A 2001 Integrated Medicine. BMJ 322(7279):119–120

Russell JK 1994 Bodywork – the art of touch. Nurse Practitioner Forum 5(2): 85–90

Ryden E 2001 Just war and pacificism: Chinese and Christian perspectives in dialogue. Ricci Institute, Taipei

Sackett DL, Rosenberg WMC, Gray JAM et al 1996 Evidence based medicine: what it is and what it isn't. BMJ 312:71–72

Smith FF 1990 Inner bridges: a guide to energy movement and body structure. Humanics, Atlanta, GA

Stone J 2002 An ethical framework for complementary and alternative therapists. Routledge, London

Tavares M 1998 An exploratory study on the use of massage and counselling skills, specifically visualisation, in chronic illness. MSc dissertation, Brunel University, Middlesex

Tavares M 2003 National guidelines for the use of complementary therapies in supportive and palliative care. The Prince's Foundation for Integrated Health, National Council for Hospice and Specialist Palliative Care Services, London

Tavares M 2005 Guide for writing policies, procedures and protocols, 2nd edn. Complementary therapies in supportive and palliative care. Help the Hospices, Hospice Information, London

Thomas K 2004 Lecture on 'Gold Standards Framework' at the 4th Annual Worcestershire Palliative Care Conference, Worcester, 24 February 2004

Twycross R 1997 Introducing palliative care, 2nd edn. Radcliffe Medical Press, Oxford

Westland G 1993 Massage as a therapeutic tool, Part 1. Journal of Occupational Therapy 56(4):129–134

FURTHER READING

Barraclough M (ed) 2001 Integrated cancer care – holistic, complementary and creative approaches. Oxford University Press, Oxford

Cooper J (ed) 1997 Occupational therapy in oncology and palliative care. Whurr Publishers Ltd, London

Cummings I 1998 The interdisciplinary team. In: Doyle D, Hanks GWC, MacDonald N (eds) Oxford Textbook of Palliative Medicine, 2nd edn. Oxford University Press, Oxford

Fulton CL, Else R 1998 Physiotherapy. In: Doyle D, Hanks GWC, MacDonald N (eds) 1998 Oxford Textbook of Palliative Medicine, 2nd edn. Oxford University Press, Oxford, pp. 819–828

Munroe B 1998 Social work in palliative care. In: Doyle D, Hanks GWC, MacDonald N (eds) Oxford Textbook of Palliative Medicine, 2nd edn. Oxford University Press, Oxford

Pearce C, Lugton J 1999 Holistic assessment of patients' and relatives' needs. In: Lugton J, Kindlen M (eds) Palliative care: the nursing role. Churchill Livingstone, Edinburgh

Speck P 1998 Spiritual issues in palliative care. In: Doyle D, Hanks GWC, MacDonald N (eds) Oxford Textbook of Palliative Medicine, 2nd edn. Oxford University Press, Oxford

Tigges KN 1998 Occupational therapy. In: Doyle D, Hanks GWC, MacDonald N (eds) Oxford Textbook of Palliative Medicine, 2nd edn. Oxford University Press, Oxford, pp. 829–837

USEFUL ADDRESSES

The Prince's Foundation for Integrated Health
33–41 Dallington Street
London, EC1V OBB
UK
Tel: 020 3119 3100
Fax: 020 3119 3101
E-mail: info@fih.org.uk

Complementary Therapies Medical Advisor
Macmillan Cancer Relief
89 Albert Embankment
London SE1 7UQ
UK

Marianne Tavares
Complementary Therapies Coordinator
St Gemma's Hospice
329 Harrogate Road
Leeds LS17 6QD
UK
Tel: 0113 218 5567

National Association of Complementary Therapists in Hospice and Palliative
    Care (NACTHPC)
Chair – Marianne Tavares
329 Harrogate Road
Leeds LS17 6QD
UK
Tel: 0113 218 5567
E-mail: mariannetavares@hotmail.com

Evaluating the evidence

3

Jacqui Stringer and Peter A Mackereth

Abstract

This chapter examines the evidence in massage and bodywork, and provides examples of recently published research. Importantly the focus of the work will be an exploration of key issues that arise when considering conducting research involving people affected by cancer. The authors are both experienced researchers and have conducted studies examining the benefits of massage and bodywork modalities in supportive and palliative care. The chapter includes possible methodologies and recommendations for raising research awareness and involvement among therapists.

KEYWORDS

evidence, funding, questions, methodologies, research work

INTRODUCTION

Massage in its many forms is experiencing both a renaissance and a reassessment as a life enhancing healthcare intervention. Increasingly the public and healthcare professionals are questioning whether or not complementary therapies should be available to patients. The lack of research evidence is often cited as a reason for not providing these therapies within conventional healthcare settings (Graham et al 1998). Whether an intervention is offered privately, through a charity or is exchequer funded, it is equally important to ascertain potential benefits, risks and costs to inform and enable service users and providers in decision making. Anecdotal reports of benefit or an intuitive belief in the therapy may be sufficient for the paying consumer; however, they are inadequate if the purchaser is accountable to the public for how healthcare money is spent.

The demand for objective evidence of benefit is not only confined to purchasers. Increasingly students, practitioners and teachers of therapies also want to have evidence and quality information with which to review their professional practice. The concept of the 'expert patient' is also emerging as patients seek health-related information and research on both complementary and conventional treatments. Societies and support groups for people with health problems often include in websites, newsletters and booklets details of the latest research, as well as individual accounts of treatment and therapy experience.

The House of Lords Science and Technology Report (2000) recommended that the complementary and alternative medicine (CAM) professions should work towards ensuring that therapeutic claims for their treatments be supported by quality evidence of benefit and safety. The report divided the most popular therapies into three categories. Group 1 included acupuncture, osteopathy and homeopathy; these were judged to have a growing body of evidence supporting therapeutic claims, as well as good progression in terms of professional regulation and training. Massage, aromatherapy and reflexology were examples of therapies classified as Group 2. The report acknowledged the popularity of these therapies with the public, but recommended greater development in regulatory structures, training and a stronger evidence base for practice. It was also recommended that training schools have greater liaison with higher education and a more robust infrastructure for research awareness and activities. Finally, Group 3, which included the practice of iridology and dowsing were deemed to have poor evidence and questionable theoretical basis.

ARGUMENTS FOR AND AGAINST ENGAGING IN RESEARCH

Knowledge can be derived from a variety of sources, which include tradition, authority, trial and error, reasoning and scientific investigation. Massage and other forms of bodywork have existed for thousands of years and will probably continue to remain popular irrespective of demands for quantifiable evidence. Charismatic and enthusiastic teachers of a therapy can have a lasting influence on how it is practised. A claim frequently made by therapists is that the benefits of massage and bodywork are numerous and often individual. Here we have two areas for debate and potential investigation already:

- It can be reasoned that the formal research process is an unnecessary, expensive and time-consuming process, when therapists, teachers and often consumers alike believe that the treatment works.
- It can be argued that reflecting on individual case studies is a process of investigation that can be used to inform our understanding of benefits, safety issues and requirements for therapist development.

Individual case studies are a useful source of information which may appear in the writings of teachers and therapists as well as individual accounts by clients who have been moved to write their own books or narratives in magazine and newspaper articles. This form of anecdotal evidence can be analysed and explored, contributing to a growing body of experience and understanding of massage and bodywork. Importantly, individual accounts are also included throughout this book to illustrate practical application and to share the positive and problematic experiences of both patients and therapists. However, this form of evidence can be subjective and difficult to replicate or quantify, given such variables as the individualised nature of the therapeutic relationship, treatment used and patient presentation. Research work using a variety of data sources, if skilfully conducted, can provide rich opportunities to examine established theory and practice and inform assumptions made about therapeutic outcomes. Potential areas for research in massage and bodywork are listed in Box 3.1.

Box 3.1
Potential areas for research

- Evidence of safety, efficacy and outcomes for people affected by cancer.
- Provide information about access and provision of massage and bodywork in conventional healthcare settings.
- Risk assessment, for example identifying contraindications or areas of caution.
- Comparative work.
- Mechanism of action.
- Assessment of patient satisfaction.
- Ascertaining research skills among practitioners and teachers.
- Evaluation of educational provision for practitioners.
- Profiling professional activities of practitioners.
- Document historical development of the practice of massage and bodywork in cancer care.

HIERARCHY OF EVIDENCE

The field of research is vast and complex, with an array of methodologies and philosophical approaches to the activity. The language used can intimidate and exclude therapists and the novice researcher. Texts and articles containing terms such as 'grounded theory', 'quasi-experimental' and 'meta-analysis' can be very confusing. However, it is important to understand the terminology as citing only the findings of research is not enough to justify the use of a particular therapy; critics will want to know the detail. For example: What was the sample size? Was there a control group? Who conducted the study (i.e. do the researchers have a track record of quality research work and supervision)? Can the findings be generalised or are they only relevant to a particular population? The methodological approach, the techniques and tools used to collect data should also be scrutinised and critiqued.

A debate exists among researchers as to which study designs are appropriate or even essential to determine efficacy. Many scientists and healthcare practitioners accept only one methodology or have a hierarchy in mind when reviewing research work, with the best evidence supposedly coming from the systematic review. To conduct the review requires investigators collecting together existing research work, critically evaluating the studies, summarising the evidence and identifying limitations. A reviewer will select studies according to inclusion criteria, for example they must have been published within a predetermined time period (say the last 10 years), involve randomisation procedures and exclude studies with less than 10 subjects per group. Unfortunately, reviews can be inconclusive, particularly if the studies were poorly conducted and reported. However, a review may identify good quality work and make recommendations for future research work.

Conventional medicine holds the randomised controlled trial (RCT) as the most acceptable form of evidence to evaluate an intervention. RCTs involve subjects being randomised to one of two or more arms of a study in which they receive different interventions; ideally both the subject and the evaluator are 'blinded' as to which intervention was received. In practice this can only really be done in pharmaceutical trials where, for example, a standard drug therapy or look-alike placebo can be compared with a new drug. A more pragmatic approach, particularly in relation to massage and bodywork research, is to use the format of an RCT where the intervention is employed in the experimental group compared with a well-matched control group that receives a conventional treatment or nothing. Subjects, although not blinded, can be randomised to the different treatment/usual care arm of the trial. For example, to evaluate the potential of reflexology to reduce anxiety, a trial could be conducted where group A receives six sessions of reflexology plus standard care (i.e. usual prescribed anxiolytics and support from healthcare professionals), whereas group B receives standard care only. Although the RCT is acknowledged in healthcare settings as the 'gold standard' for evidence-based care, this is beginning to change. Ernst (2001) recommends that the optimal methodology is one that best answers the question being posed. Examples of suggested questions and methodologies can be seen in Table 3.1.

SOURCES OF INFORMATION

It has been argued that therapists should know how to access the research literature, be able to constructively critique research papers, and most importantly for patient work, be able to 'interpret the practical implications' (Vickers 1995, p. 143) of any findings. Inaccessibility of research papers and the lack of appraisal skills can be major stumbling blocks to the dissemination of best evidence to the practice arena. It is important to acknowledge that while research work on massage and bodywork in cancer care is newly developing, evidence does exist supporting the value of massage in a wide range of health problems. Computerised databases can be a useful starting point for locating research papers that may be of interest. Increasingly, the Internet, via search

Table 3.1
Optimal study designs for different research questions

Examples of research questions	Appropriate methods/design
Proving	
'Is there a specific beneficial effect of massage in cancer care?' (Efficacy)	Explanatory RCT Quasi-experimental design
'How well does providing reflexology for nausea work in practice?' (Effectiveness)	Outcome studies
Improving	
'Is hara analysis a useful diagnostic test?' (Developmental studies)	Comparative study
Picturing	
'Who uses aromatherapy in cancer care and why?'	Population survey Purchaser and provider surveys
'Who provides lymphoedema massage and why?' (Snapshots)	Focus groups and interviews
Understanding	
'How does aromatherapy work to combat MRSA infection?' (Basic clinical research)	Laboratory research Explanatory RCT Quasi-experimental design Case studies
Developing research tools	
'How do we assess the processes and effects of chair massage for carers?' (Outcome measures and instrumentation)	Development and validation of measures and instruments Cohort studies

Adapted from Foundation for Integrated Medicine (1997).
MRSA, methicillin resistant *Staphylococcus aureus*; RCT, randomised controlled trial.

engines, can be used to find published studies, although this information can be incorrect and lack detail. For example a review of websites on CAM and cancer by Schmidt and Ernst (2004) concluded that the information and claims made on many websites were misleading and unsubstantiated.

Possibly the best source for quality research is the peer-reviewed journal or books by authors/teams of authors with a track record of high quality work.

One team of researchers stands out in its contribution to understanding the power of touch. The team is led by Dr Tiffany Field at the Touch Research Institutes (TRI) in Miami, FL, USA (Mackereth 2001). This team has shown, for example, that massage can improve various parameters of immune function, psychological measures and disease markers. Peer-reviewed journals usually include an abstract at the beginning of each paper, which provides an overview of the study, but rarely gives sufficient information to decide whether the study was conducted properly. There is a skill in reading and reviewing published papers, but unfortunately it is not usually covered in a therapist's training. Kahn (2001), a teacher of massage, states that training schools have an important role in transforming massage therapists into a research-conscious profession, for example by enabling students to access peer-reviewed journals, providing guidance on literature review, teaching sessions on research methodology and how to critique studies, as well as evidence-based teaching. Opportunities to access research expertise are increasingly occurring with massage schools either linked via accreditation systems or with touch therapy courses offered in university settings. Undergraduates studying massage can not only expand their educational experience and access to resources, but may also be encouraged to consider postgraduate studies and research work. These developments can have a snowball effect on improving the quality and numbers of research projects, and if published, further increase the available literature.

THE PROCESS AND CHALLENGE OF RESEARCH WORK

The research process begins with the identification and clarification of the area of research. This has to be more focused than just wanting to research massage and bodywork or to prove that it is beneficial for all. It is important for any budding researcher to consider the relevance and the feasibility of a proposed project and for this reason it is helpful to gain the support of an experienced researcher. If, for example, the study aims to show enhanced wellbeing of patients, a potential problem might be in recruiting sufficient numbers to adequately demonstrate an effect.

The researcher might develop an excellent project, yet lack the finances to undertake it. Although CAM research activity has grown over the last decade, funding continues to be one of the greatest challenges to overcome alongside lack of research awareness. Goethe's last words were 'More light', but who pays the light bill for research? There are costs involved with any research activity, including paying for a researcher's time, fees for statistical advice, charges for registering to use outcome measures and costs associated with data collection, e.g. postage. There are ways of raising the funds internally from professional bodies representing a therapy or through the institution employing the therapist/researcher or by applying to charities affiliated with that institution. Research projects requiring external funding must find a willing and interested body to convince, and any researcher applying for funding from a particular organisation must address their application to its mission statement. An encouraging development in the UK, following calls for greater CAM research, has been for the government to fund a rolling programme of fellowships linked to the university sector with the intention of building research expertise and evidence in the CAM field (Ernst et al 2005).

It is important to recognise that a published research paper can range from the results of a brief audit to the culmination of up to 5 years' work – as is the case in a part-time PhD. The PhD process will have involved development and clarification of the research question, reviewing the relevant literature, identification of a suitable research design and appropriate outcome measures, painstaking data collection, analysis and report writing. Following graduation the successful PhD candidate usually prepares reports of the work that match the requirements and readership interests of a peer-reviewed journal. Whether the project is large or small, there are basic issues which apply to all, and some simple suggestions for the budding researcher are given in Box 3.2.

Importantly, an interest in research does not necessarily mean instigating and leading a project but it can involve joining a research interest group,

Box 3.2
Getting started in research

A summary of suggested steps is as follows:

- Start small and simple by focusing on a single question, CAM intervention and target population.
- Make sure your research question is clear and concise.
- Do not try to fit your question to a pre-conceived idea of what your study design should be, read the literature and explore your choices.
- Get support from someone with research experience, for example contact your local university for research contacts and courses.
- Consider investigating possible sources of funding – the university research contact may also be able to advise here.
- Ask your professional body about research interest groups and support for your project.
- Ensure that the practice being researched reflects normal practice, i.e. used by therapists who are experienced. Devise protocols that encompass best practice rather than constrain it.
- Consider the ethical issues involved in the project, for example consent and access issues and concerns about the vulnerability of patients.
- Limit sources of bias in the project, for example making sure the therapist(s) and data collector(s) are not the same person/people.
- All research studies require ethical approval. Find someone with experience to help with your application.

subscribing to peer-reviewed journals, being a therapist for a research study or enrolling to being a research subject.

RECENT RESEARCH WORK

There is now a growing body of research relating to massage for patients living with cancer. In Table 3.2 a summary of some recent research in massage and bodywork in cancer care has been compiled; although this is not a systematic review it does provide an overview of each project. Some of these studies, evaluating the use of massage, aromatherapy and reflexology in cancer care, are now briefly discussed in terms of methodology and findings. Care has to be taken in interpreting reports of significant differences between groups or treatment arms, as findings may not be either generalisable to a wider population or clinically significant.

Massage

As an example of a large-scale study, Cassileth and Vickers (2004) reported effects of massage on over 1000 cancer patients from the Sloan–Kettering Cancer Center over a period of 3 years. They concluded that massage had an immediate and substantive beneficial effect by reducing symptoms of anxiety, depression, pain and nausea. They also reported that in the case of outpatients these benefits were still evident at least 48 hours later. In another large study, again with cancer patients, Post-White et al (2003) showed massage reduced ratings in several measures including anxiety and perception of pain in 230 patients. From a slightly different perspective, cancer patients have also been seen to be proactive in using complementary therapies – including massage – to both improve immune function and ameliorate the side effects of cancer treatments. Morris et al (2000), in a postal survey enquiring about use of complementary therapies, received a total of 617 replies from the original 1935 questionnaires sent to a random selection of cancer patients attending their centre. They discovered that 53% of these patients used massage, and that this was one of the top three therapies used (the others being nutrition therapy (63%) and healing herbs (44%)).

A clinical study by Ahles et al (1999) showed that in patients (n = 35) undergoing an autologous bone marrow transplant as part of their cancer treatment, massage led to significant reduction in diastolic blood pressure, nausea, distress and anxiety, particularly in the time period directly following the massage. Equally, Smith et al (2003) looked at specific healing outcomes following a series of one of three different interventions (massage, therapeutic touch or 'friendly visit') for patients (n = 88) undergoing bone marrow transplantation. They showed, using a rating scale developed by the researchers, that there were a number of perceived benefits from massage therapy, including reduced scores in, for example, insomnia and anxiety and/or depression. In this study subjects were seen every third day for the duration of their continuation in the study (criteria for discharge not stated) both as inpatients

Table 3.2
Examples of recent research work 1999–2004

Study	Purpose/Condition	Method	Treatment/ Groups	Outcome measures	Findings	Commentary
Ahles et al (1999)	To assess the impact of massage in patients undergoing bone marrow transplantation	Randomised controlled study (n = 35)	(1) Up to nine 20-minute sessions of massage (n = 16) (2) Standard treatment (n = 18)	STAI, BPI, POMS, SAI Numerical scales of distress, fatigue, nausea and pain HR, BP, RR	Massage group scored significantly lower on the mid-treatment SAI Both groups showed significant decline with time on scores from POMS and trait anxiety	Small number of subjects Amount of massage received not standardised
Wilkinson et al (1999)	An evaluation of aromatherapy massage in palliative care	Randomised controlled study (n = 103)	Massage with or without aromatherapy (Roman camomile essential oil)	STAI Rotterdam Symptom checklist Semi-structured interview	Massage with or without aromatherapy reduced levels of anxiety Significant improvement in quality of life with the addition of aromatherapy	Attrition rate was high; 16 left the study due to deterioration in condition or death Patients' condition variable across the group No double-blind features so therapists knew they were administering aromatherapy

Table 3.2 continued over

Table 3.2
Examples of recent research work 1999–2004—cont'd

Study	Purpose/Condition	Method	Treatment/ Groups	Outcome measures	Findings	Commentary
Field (2000)	Effects of massage on women with breast cancer	Randomised control study (n = 20)	30-minute body massage twice a week for 5 weeks (n = 10) Control group (n = 10)	STAI, POMS, FLI Pain questionnaire (SF-MPQ) Symptom checklist Immune and biochemical measures	Significant reduction by group in anxiety and depression Significant increase in immune function	Short duration of the study – unable to assess effects on cancer remission
Grealish et al (2000)	To assess the effects of foot massage on nausea, pain and relaxation in hospitalised patients with cancer	Cross-over randomised controlled trial (n = 87)	(1) Two sessions of foot massage and (2) Quiet time	HR Pain (VAS) Nausea (VAS) Self-report of relaxation (VAS)	Significant difference in all measures Improving relaxation and reducing nausea and pain	No control for medication No exploration of lasting effects Numbers in each group not given 10-minute sessions only Therapists were trained reflexologists

	Aim	Method			Results	Comments
Morris et al (2000)	Characterisation of the use of complementary therapies in breast cancer patients versus patients with cancer in other primary sites	Survey (n = 617) (288 breast cancer patients and 329 other)	Initial mailing of questionnaires done to 935 patients with breast cancer and 1000 patients with other primary site diagnoses	N/A	Most commonly used therapies were: nutrition (63%) massage (53%) healing herbs (44%)	Useful information gleaned relating to the use of complementary therapies and the reasons for usage
Dunwoody et al 2002	To understand the personal meaning of aromatherapy to patients with cancer	Quantitative (n = 11)	Focus group interview	N/A	Identification of eight themes including de-stressing effects of aromatherapy, patient empowerment and communication through touch	
Stephenson et al (2000)	To assess the effects of reflexology on pain and anxiety in patients with lung and breast cancers	Quasi-experimental cross-over trial (n = 23)	(1) Reflexology (2) No intervention period	Pain (SF-MPQ) Anxiety (VAS)	Significant decrease in anxiety following reflexology in both groups Significant decrease in pain in breast cancer group	Only 2 out of the 10 lung cancer patients reported pain compared with 11 out of 13 in the breast cancer group. Gender differences between the groups and effects of pain relief makes it difficult to interpret results

Table 3.2 continued over

Table 3.2
Examples of recent research work 1999–2004—cont'd

Study	Purpose/Condition	Method	Treatment/ Groups	Outcome measures	Findings	Commentary
Lively et al (2002)	An economic evaluation of the cost savings of massage therapy in alleviating high-dose chemotherapy-induced nausea and vomiting	(n = 31) 14 controls received anti-emetics, 17 received massage as an adjunct to anti-emetics	Thrice weekly massage sessions with 50% of patients receiving a maximum of five treatments	Record of days with: nausea and vomiting, total parenteral nutrition, control with anti-emetic in treatment programme	The use of massage therapy in the 17 patients resulted in significant cost savings ($2853.10 per patient)	Small sample size Only one therapist used Nursing costs not included One chemotherapy regimen assessed Did not quantify effects on anxiety or stress
Gambles et al (2002)	An evaluation of a hospice-based reflexology service	Qualitative study (n = 34)	Semi-structure questionnaire	Thematic analysis of the questionnaire data	Positive comments; improved wellbeing, comfort support, able to cope with symptoms and treatment	Hospice staff and therapist distributed the questionnaire No demographic details Sensitive approach taken given the vulnerability of service users in this setting
Smith (2002)	Evaluation of reflexology for patients with breast cancer undergoing radiotherapy	Randomised controlled trial (n = 150)	(1) Reflexology (2) Foot massage (3) Standard care only	POMS, Pearson-Byars Fatigue check-list, lymphocyte activity	Significant differences for foot massage compared with standard care group in some subscale of the POMS and Fatigue checklist Trend for a possible effect on lymphocyte activity in reflexology group	Researcher also practitioner Used foot massage as a sham treatment

Post-White et al (2003)	To evaluate the effectiveness of massage (MT), healing touch (HT) and caring presence (P) in reducing the side effects of cancer treatment	Randomised, prospective, cross-over intervention study (n = 230)	Four weekly 45-minute sessions of assigned intervention plus 4 weekly sessions of standard care (control) – order of sessions was randomised. After 4 sessions in one condition they received 4 sessions in the other condition	HR, RR, BP, one item score (0–10) of current pain and current nausea, BPI, POMS, assessment of analgesic and anti-emetic use, satisfaction with care through self-devised questionnaires	MT and HT are more effective than P alone or standard care at reducing pain, fatigue and mood disturbance in patients with cancer receiving chemotherapy	29% attrition rate; 164 patients completed all eight sessions. Question-mark over appropriateness of study design in such poorly patients
Smith et al (2003)	To investigate the effects of therapeutic touch (TT) and massage therapy (MT) on various outcome measures relating to bone marrow transplantation	Randomised clinical trial (n = 88)	(1) Standardised TT every third day (2) Standardised MT every third day (3) Friendly visit (FV) every third day	Time to engraftment. Complications. Patient perceptions of benefit of therapy	MT significantly lowered scores for nervous system/neurological complications compared with control group. Patients' perceptions of benefits of MT were also significantly higher than for FV	High attrition rate. No standard massage protocol. FV provided by an untrained volunteer

Table 3.2 continued over

Table 3.2
Examples of recent research work 1999–2004—cont'd

Study	Purpose/Condition	Method	Treatment/Groups	Outcome measures	Findings	Commentary
Hernandez-Reif et al (2004)	To assess the effects of massage on the immune system, neuroendocrine system and perceived stress in women with early stages of breast cancer	Randomised controlled trial (n = 34)	(1) Five weeks of massage (15 sessions) (2) Standard medical care	STAI, POMS, SCL-90-R, Life events questionnaire, NK cells, lymphocytes, catecholamines	Massage group showed: short-term reduced anxiety, depressed mood and anger; longer-term reduction of depression and hostility; increased dopamine, serotonin, NK cells and lymphocytes	Small sample Only assessed changes over 5 weeks – need for longitudinal study Randomisation 'flip of the coin'
Cassileth & Vickers (2004)	Change in cancer-related symptom scores from pre- to post-massage therapy	Survey (n = 1290)	Analysis of data from symptom cards (which used rating scales)	Rating scales relating to several symptoms including: pain, fatigue, nausea and depression	Symptoms scores were reduced in approximately 50% of patients Benefits persisted – especially in outpatients	Large variation in patients, for example some were inpatients and some were outpatients

Abbreviations: SAI, State Anxiety Inventory; STAI, State Trait Anxiety Inventory; BNI, Brief Nausea Index; BPI, Brief Pain Inventory; HR, heart rate; VAS, visual analogue scale; FLI, Functional Living Index – Cancer Scale; SF-MPQ, short-form McGill Pain Questionnaire; SCL-90-R, symptom checklist; POMS, Profile of Mood States; NK, natural killer; RR, respiratory rate.

and outpatients. The number of sessions received by each subject was not standardised. Unfortunately, 27 withdrew (25 of these withdrew following assignment to study arm), suggesting an element of discomfort with the protocol.

Hernandez-Reif and colleagues (2004) have recently completed a study looking at improving mood, immune function and reducing levels of stress through massage in 34 women with early stage (I and II) breast cancer. Their results suggest massage to be beneficial in a number of ways, including significant reductions in anxiety and depression scores ($p < 0.05$) and enhancement of immune function through increase in numbers of natural killer (NK) cells in the massage group ($p < 0.05$). An analysis of co-variance performed on numbers of NK cells from first to last day of the 5-week study period disclosed a significant group effect ($p < 0.05$). This reflected a significant positive change ($p < 0.05$) in NK cell numbers for the massage arm and a negative change for the control arm.

Aromatherapy

Wilkinson et al (1999), in their work with cancer patients in a hospice setting, suggested that the benefits of massage are greater when essential oils are used, although not necessarily to the point of significance. They randomised 103 patients to receive a series of three hour-long weekly massages, either with base oil or with aromatherapy oil. This team observed a number of significant improvements in both physiological and psychological subscales for patients in both intervention arms. The authors noted that improvements appeared to be greater for patients in the aromatherapy arm although they suggested this may be partly due to the nurse therapists behaving differently with patients in the aromatherapy arm. In an attempt to understand what receiving aromatherapy massage meant to cancer patients, Dunwoody et al (2002) explored the qualitative aspects of receiving massage using an interview technique with 11 oncology outpatients in the setting of a focus group. In this work aromatherapy massage was carried out in a clinically appropriate way with the therapist and patient choosing the oils for the massage together. Dunwoody et al's results confirmed the de-stressing effects of massage as well as highlighting other benefits such as empowerment of the patient.

Reflexology

In the UK, Gambles et al (2002) sought to gather 'user' perspectives by using a semi-structured questionnaire with a convenience sample of patients (n = 34) attending for between four and six reflexology treatments at a hospice. Patient feedback was overwhelmingly positive, with accounts of relief from tension and anxiety, feelings of comfort and support from the therapists and improved wellbeing. Many of the patients identified the treatment with being better able to cope with their diagnosis and conventional treatment. The use of a short questionnaire, just six items, was argued on the basis of not burdening this vulnerable patient group. The hospice staff and therapist gave out the questionnaire, which may have biased the responses.

A quasi-experimental design was used to establish the effects of foot massage provided by nurse therapists (Grealish et al 2000). A total of 87 hospitalised patients with cancer were randomised to three protocols of massage and one quiet period resting on their beds. After their first treatment they then either received a second massage or rested. The third treatment was again either resting or massage. In effect the three protocols required patients to receive two massages and one resting period, but in different order. Visual analogue scales were used to measure pain, nausea and relaxation. Significant differences were found following the massage interventions, with scores demonstrating improved relaxation and reduced nausea and pain. The nurses providing the massage were reported as being trained reflexologists, but the treatment given and how patients were randomised were not described in detail.

In the USA, Stephenson et al (2000) conducted a quasi-experimental study utilising a cross-over design. Inpatients (n = 23) with lung or breast cancer were randomised to receive (1) 30 minutes of reflexology followed by a 30-minute control time after a 2-day break or (2) 30 minutes of control time, 2-day break and then 30 minutes of reflexology. There was a significant decrease in anxiety observed in patients following the reflexology intervention, but effects on pain reduction were less clear. Gender differences in the groups and the effects of pain medication made it difficult to interpret the results. One of the advantages of the design was that all patients received the same interventions/control but at different time intervals. Stephenson not only collected the data but also provided all the reflexology treatments, which may have influenced the responses to the self-report measures used. One treatment alone is not usual reflexology practice so there is a need to evaluate a series of treatments and perhaps compare outcomes with another CAM intervention in a larger sample.

In a PhD thesis study by Smith (2002), a radiographer and reflexologist, sought to evaluate the effects of reflexology on fatigue, mood and lymphocyte activity in a group of women (n = 150) with breast cancer undergoing radiotherapy. There were significant differences for foot massage (n = 47) and reflexology (n = 44) groups when compared with the standard care group (n = 38) in some of the Profile of Mood States subscales and the Pearson–Byars Fatigue Feeling Checklist, and a trend only for a possible effect on lymphocyte activity in the reflexology group. The researcher regretted not including a means of collecting qualitative data, given that informally many participants reported a range of benefits from both interventions. As funding was limited, Smith provided both the reflexology and sham (foot massage) treatments, with only four sessions possible. A total of 21 patients were lost to the study, with five withdrawn by the researcher for health reasons. In the standard care group, 12 failed to complete the questionnaires. Smith also acknowledged that foot massage was not a satisfactory sham treatment given that reflex areas of the feet were massaged in the process.

What these studies show is that there are many examples of studies using a variety of methodologies, which are available for potential researchers to review prior to making decisions relating to their own work. It is important to fit the methodology of the study to the research question rather than to try to manipulate the research question into a certain pre-conceived 'best' study design.

SUMMARY

For practitioners of massage and bodywork, the idea of being involved or leading a research project may well be an overwhelming challenge. However, if certain guidelines are followed and support available, research is manageable and can greatly inform clinical practice. In this chapter recommendations have been made for the budding researcher, but an important starting point is developing an appreciation and awareness of the growing body of research evidence. Research is an important source of information about massage and bodywork practice, but it needs to be relevant and useful to patients, therapists and future researchers, as well as for those funding services in cancer care. As the expertise in CAM research grows, there is a great potential for the experience and effects of skilful touch in cancer care to be illuminated and shared with both the public and health professionals.

REFERENCES

Ahles TA, Tope DM, Pinkson B et al 1999 Massage therapy for patients undergoing autologous bone marrow transplantation. Journal of Pain and Symptom Management 18(3):157–163

Cassileth BR, Vickers AJ 2004 Massage therapy for symptom control: outcome study at a major cancer centre. Journal of Pain and Symptom Management 28(3):244–249

Dunwoody L, Smyth A, Davidson R 2002 Cancer patients' experiences and evaluations of aromatherapy massage in palliative care. International Journal of Palliative Nursing 8(10):497–504

Ernst E 2001 Evidence-based massage therapy: a contradiction in terms. In: Rich GJ (ed) Massage therapy: the evidence for practice. Harcourt Brace, London

Ernst E, Schmidt K, Wilder B 2005 CAM research in Britain: the last 10 years. Complementary Therapies in Clinical Practice 11:17–20

Field T 2000 Touch therapy. Harcourt Press, London

Foundation for Integrated Medicine 1997 Integrated healthcare: a way forward for the next five years? Foundation for Integrated Medicine, London

Gambles M, Crooke M, Wilkinson S 2002 Evaluation of a hospice based reflexology service: a qualitative audit of patient perceptions. European Journal of Oncology Nursing 6(1):37–44

Graham L, Goldstone L, Eijundu A et al 1998 Penetration of complementary therapies into NHS trust and private hospital practice. Complementary Therapies in Nursing and Midwifery 4(6):160–165

Grealish L, Lomasney A, Whiteman B 2000 Foot massage: a nursing intervention to modify the distressing symptoms of pain and nausea in patients hospitalised with cancer. Cancer Nursing 23(3):237–243

Hernandez-Reif M, Ironson G, Field T 2004 Breast cancer patients have improved immune and neuroendocrine functions following massage therapy. Journal of Psychosomatic Research 57:45–52

House of Lords Select Committee on Science and Technology Sixth Report 2000 Complementary and Alternative Medicine. The Stationery Office, London

Kahn J 2001 Research matters. Massage Magazine Issue 92 July/August

Lively BT, Holiday-Goodman M, Black C et al 2002 Massage therapy for chemotherapy-induced emesis. In: Rich GJ (ed) Massage therapy: the evidence for practice. Harcourt Brace, London

Mackereth P 2001 Touch Research Institutes; an interview with Dr Tiffany Field. Complementary Therapies in Nursing and Midwifery 7:84–89

Morris KT, Johnson N, Homer L et al 2000 A comparison of complementary therapy use between breast cancer patients and patients with other primary tumour sites. American Journal of Surgery 179:407–411

Post-White J, Kinney ME, Savik MS et al 2003 Therapeutic massage and healing touch improve symptoms in cancer. Integrative Cancer Therapies 2(4): 332–344

Schmidt K, Ernst E 2004 Assessing websites on complementary and alternative medicine for cancer. Annals of Oncology 15:733–742

Smith MC, Reeder F, Daniel L et al 2003 Outcomes of touch therapies during bone marrow transplant. Alternative Therapies 9(1):40–49

Smith G 2002 A randomised controlled clinical trial of reflexology in breast cancer patients, to reduce fatigue resulting from radiotherapy to the breast and chest wall. PhD thesis, University of Liverpool, Liverpool (unpublished)

Stephenson NLN, Weinrich SP 2000 The effects of foot reflexology on anxiety and pain in patients with breast and lung cancer. Oncology Nursing Forum 27(1):67–72

Vickers A 1995 A basic introduction to medical research. Part 3: what can the practitioner do? Complementary Therapies in Nursing and Midwifery 1: 143–147

Wilkinson S, Aldridge J, Salmon I et al 1999 An evaluation of aromatherapy massage in palliative care. Palliative Medicine 13(5):409–417

FURTHER READING

Batavia M 2001 Clinical research for health professionals. Butterworth-Heinemann, Oxford

Freeman LW, Lawlis GF (eds) 2001 Complementary and alternative medicine: a research-based approach. Mosby, London

Rich G (ed) 2000 Massage therapy: the evidence for practice. Harcourt Brace, London

USEFUL ADDRESS

Jacqui Stringer
Clinical Lead Complementary Therapy Service
c/o The Adult Leukaemia Unit
Christie Hospital
Wilmslow Road
Manchester M20 4BX
UK
E-mail: Jacqui.stringer@christie-tr.nwest.nhs.uk

Website of Touch Research Institutes: http://www.miami.edu/touch-research/
    triresearch.htm

4

Professional and potent practice

Peter A Mackereth and Ann Carter

Abstract

This chapter focuses on the issues and challenges experienced by therapists working with people affected by cancer. The discussion is centred on the characteristics of a profession as proposed by Houle in 1980 and explored in the context of the '3 Ps' (permission, protection and potency) model of practice developed by Crossman in 1966. Included in the content are strategies to support and encourage reflective practice, such as continuing education activities and clinical supervision. The purpose of including this chapter in this book is to emphasise the importance of professional practice for massage and bodywork therapists in cancer care.

KEYWORDS

professionalism, accountability, reflective practice, safety, mentoring and leadership

INTRODUCTION

An important question to ask is, 'Why choose to work with massage and bodywork in a cancer care setting?'. There are many complex and curious reasons why a career or vocational path in massage and bodywork therapies is followed. For some it might be an activity that is purely voluntary, for others it is a development of their existing role as a health professional. Others may find themselves in remunerated positions, either as a sessional therapist or in a part-time contracted position. Whatever the arrangements, the work is focused on supporting patients and carers who are facing the challenge of a life-threatening illness. The reasons for working with people living with cancer can vary, and may be linked to a personal experience of cancer (see Box 4.1). When therapists choose to work in this setting, they face many challenges in very diverse areas. These challenges include adapting treatments, interacting with patients, carers and health professionals in a medical setting, as well as handling the physical, emotional and spiritual aspects of the illness. In

Box 4.1
Therapist's narrative

I started training in massage and reflexology during the last few years of my mother's life. She had been having bleeds and was being investigated while I was working in a cytology laboratory. Knowing what I knew, I suspected it was cancer, and the results confirmed this. The prognosis was poor and I wanted to have quality time with my mother. I was so pleased to be able to provide short treatments to help ease her discomfort and pain, particularly when her medications did not give enough relief.

A year later I started offering my services as a volunteer in a cancer setting. Occasionally patients' symptoms and/or how they are dealing with the cancer remind me of my mother. My colleagues have similar stories; some have had a brush with cancer themselves or lost a family member or close friend from cancer. Cancer seems to touch everyone's lives, so the experience can be a shared one.

I have attended courses related to the work and every day brings new experiences and challenges. Supervision and informal relationships developed with colleagues provide opportunities to talk, share experiences and exchange treatments.

The patients are very appreciative, both in words and in how they physically respond to the treatments. I am also aware that many are distressed from the experience of cancer and can be helped by receiving massage and other therapies, and also for some they are growing spiritually.

addition, some therapists are taking on a co-ordinating role in supportive and palliative care (Tavares 2003), which involves the management and development of a complementary therapy service.

BEING A PROFESSIONAL

The characteristics of a profession were described by Houle. Although proposed in the 1980s, Houle's model has relevance even today when examining how therapists can emerge as valued members of a multidisciplinary cancer team. It has also been suggested that a practitioner needs to bring the '3 Ps' (potency, protection and permission) to their therapeutic work (Crossman 1966). In order to explore the relationship between professional and potent practice the two models have been integrated and form the basis for exploration in this chapter (see Box 4.2).

Houle's (1980) characteristics have been grouped under the '3 Ps' as they fit usefully within this framework and the aims of this chapter. Specific characteristics are discussed in more depth relevant to massage and bodywork practice.

> **Box 4.2**
> Professional and potent practice: incorporating the work of Crossman
> (1966) and Houle (1980)
>
> **Permission**
> - Public acceptance.
> - Service to society.
> - Role distinction.
> - Ethical practice.
>
> **Protection**
> - Legal reinforcement of professional standards.
> - Penalties against incompetent or unethical practice.
> - Formal training.
> - Credentialing system to certify competence.
>
> **Potency**
> - Use of theoretical knowledge.
> - A concept of a mission, open to change.
> - Mastery of theoretical knowledge.
> - Having the capacity to solve problems.
> - Continued seeking of self-enhancement (by its members).
> - Creation of a subculture.

PERMISSION

Public (and professional) acceptance

Approximately a third of people living with cancer in the UK will seek treatments from complementary therapists outside the National Health Service (NHS), indeed many patients are now demanding access to complementary and alternative medicine (CAM) (Lewith et al 2002, White 1998). Currently, the provision of complementary therapies in the NHS is largely restricted to supportive and palliative care settings (Roberts et al 2005, Wilkinson 2002). However, a recent report on clinical governance and CAM to the Department of Health identified that there was an 'emerging landscape of opportunities' for complementary therapists to be included in the NHS mainstream (Wilkinson et al 2004, p. 1). The report, based on the University of Westminster study 'Clinical governance for complementary and alternative medicine in primary care' (Wilkinson et al 2005), mapped complementary healthcare in primary care. Evidence was gathered from 73% (n = 221) of the Primary Care Trusts in England. The study revealed that complementary treatments are being provided by lay therapists with further training (54%), as well as health professionals. Wilkinson et al (2005) recommend that where lay therapists are employed on NHS contracts good systems of registration, revalidation and local accountability (clinical governance) will be required.

Aside from public acceptance there is clearly a need for health professionals to be conversant with complementary therapies and able to informatively engage with patients with regard to both the benefits and risks. Although patients do not need 'permission' to explore therapies, it is important that they can access the best of complementary and conventional therapies. Patients require all professionals to work with their best interests in mind, but not to be paternalistic or make judgements about therapies, without being sufficiently informed. In cancer care settings an appreciation of each other's contribution can be facilitated by multidisciplinary meetings and shared learning experiences opportunities, e.g. team conferences and study days.

Service to society

On a macroscopic level, the movement to embrace complementary therapy with its emphasis on holistic care, not only challenges technological approaches to illness management but also provides choices. The hospice movement has been instrumental in providing an increasing range of complementary therapies to patients and their families (Kohn 1999). Conventional medicine has its limitations and in times of crisis or when facing a future living with chronic illness, the treatments may offer little, if any, meaningful comfort. Engaging in a massage treatment may be seen as peripheral, but it does provide a space to receive nurturing support through physical contact. It is important to acknowledge that the increased integration of complementary therapies into conventional care (particularly massage and other approaches to bodywork), is part of a larger movement of an increased public interest in health.

Role distinction

Massage and bodywork may be provided by lay therapists or one of the professions allied to medicine. Nurses, physiotherapists and other health professionals have assisted the greater integration of complementary therapies (Rankin-Box 1997, Tiran 1996). An important difficulty for a health professional is the control exerted by the medical profession and management structures, which constrain the development of allied professions to achieve greater autonomy in clinical practice (Kendrick 1999). There is a danger that a therapist, without being a formal health professional, might be viewed as someone who is delegated the task of 'doing' a massage. Equally, health professionals might perceive that obtaining a certificate in massage as enabling them to carry out the 'task' of massage, without appreciating that it is a separate and distinct professional occupation. There are also issues that arise when a massage therapist instead of supporting a distressed patient begins to engage in counselling or another intervention. Massage therapists need to work within their role, recognising professional boundaries and making appropriate referrals (see Chapter 2).

Ethical practice

Ethical principles, such as respect for autonomy, justice, avoidance of harm (non-maleficence), and beneficence (doing good) (Beauchamp & Childress 1994), underpin ethical practice. A duty of care is also central to ethical practice. Therapists, mindful of the intention to help, need to ensure that interventions are of benefit and 'do no harm'. It is therefore important that, if in doubt, do not proceed. For example, making claims such as deep tissue massage being appropriate for a patient with lymphoedema would not only be harmful (see Chapter 12) but also be making false claims, with failure to fully inform the patient about the benefits and risks of the treatment. Complementary therapists need to adhere to their codes of professional practice, be conversant with policies and guidelines, and accept responsibility and accountability for practice.

Respect for autonomy is essential in treating others with respect and is an acknowledgement of their personhood. This principle is important to ensure that patients can make informed choices, that their rights are upheld and that they are treated at all times with dignity. Where autonomy might be compromised (i.e. the patient is extremely ill) care must be exercised not to act in a paternalistic way, for example massaging a patient who is disoriented, believing it might help, without discussing and seeking permission for this activity from the patient's family and the primary health care practitioner.

PROTECTION

Legal enforcement of professional standards/penalties against incompetent or unethical practice

The arena of massage and bodywork presents a number of challenges for upholding and maintaining professional practice. Concerns arise in relation to (1) consent, (2) scope of practice, (3) malpractice and (4) false claims (Cohen 2003, Stone 2003). Currently there are a number of professional organisations that register complementary therapists, resulting in many different codes and standards of practice (Tavares 2003).

A key premise of professional practice is the concept of accountability, which means that therapists are answerable for their actions or inactions. Accountability is underpinned by a sense of responsibility towards performance of duties according to professional standards (Stone 2002). Codes of conduct also usually emphasise the importance of safety and maintaining competence. Incompetence can be a complex issue when standards vary in training and assessment, and when clinical practice has a limited research base (Dimond 1995). Stone (2002) argues that incompetent and unethical practice could include making false claims for interventions, putting a patient at risk from potentially harmful treatment or treating a patient who cannot give consent. Besides causing harm and distress, failure to adhere to a code of conduct can lead to removal from the organisation's register. More importantly, patients and/or their representatives can seek redress through the legal system. For example, if a therapist has failed to obtain consent for using touch, this could be treated as abuse. It could also include going beyond that for which the consent was originally sought. Therapists can also be held liable for acts or omissions which are negligent, i.e. where the action/inaction fails to meet the 'standard expected of a reasonable practitioner' (Stone 2002, p. 74).

Formal training and credentialing

Currently massage and bodywork practitioners are trained in several ways. These can range from courses in massage and reflexology for use in a beauty context to degrees in complementary therapy (Mackereth & O'Hara 2002). The level of knowledge and practical skills offered by courses vary widely and standardisation has been recommended in the House of Lords Report (2000), particularly for those in Group 2 (i.e. massage, reflexology and aromatherapy). Foundation courses in massage and bodywork do not appear to cover cancer in any depth, and cancer is often viewed as a definite contraindication for massage. While it is important to recognise that therapists need to stay within the boundaries of their knowledge and expertise, distress may be caused to a patient through a therapist in private practice refusing to work with them. An interpretation of this refusal can be that the disease somehow makes the person untouchable and unwanted. It would be responsible and considerate practice for therapists to explain that they have not yet had the training to work competently with patients living/diagnosed with cancer.

There is a need for foundation courses to give students accurate information and skills to ensure that they can converse sensitively and safely with patients. For example, a therapist who has experience in cancer care could be invited to talk to students as a guest speaker. This would provide an opportunity for students to access relevant and research-based literature on massage and cancer and the experiences of the therapist.

It is important for both therapists and the work that steps are taken to work in a way that protects the patient, the therapist and the organisation and also to be aware of their legal and ethical responsibilities.

POTENCY

Use of theoretical knowledge

Therapists need to have specialist knowledge over and above the content and skills gained through a foundation programme in massage and bodywork. While policies and procedures need to be in place, one challenge for therapists is to learn how to adapt their practice to support individual patient needs.

This involves an understanding of the illness and its treatments as well as the development of therapeutic skills (see Chapter 1). Important everyday tasks for a therapist working in cancer care can involve working in ways that are not conventional; indeed they could be seen as working at the edge of practice. These may include situations where a patient is receiving chemotherapy intravenously or is breathless and using oxygen therapy. Therapists may also need to adapt treatments so they can be given safely and effectively in patients' homes, or when working with a carer at the patient's bedside.

A concept of a mission

Vollmer and Mills (1966) contested that professionalisation is an ideal that occupations strive to attain, moving from the point of non-professional to professional. Being open to change is emphasised by Houle (1980) as an important characteristic of an evolving professional group. Complementary therapists often argue that their practice is holistic and evolving. Their work is claimed to be individualised and mindful of body, mind, spirit and the emotions (Daniel 2001). Is this degree of flexibility and fluidity based on science or are massage and bodywork art forms? With having a mission there is also a danger of becoming a zealot, someone whose aim is to convert rather than provide a person-centred service. Finding a balance between enthusiasm for an occupation and the ability to recognise its limitations is essential. Massage and bodywork therapies are complex interventions, in that there may be numerous factors that contribute to or even impede a therapeutic response(s). A successful outcome from one treatment for one patient does not mean that benefits can be assumed for a wider population. In working in cancer care, the issue of a mission is also fraught with a desire to help others who may or may not survive the disease. Massage and bodywork does not claim to cure; its mission could be to help alleviate symptoms, improve wellbeing, comfort and support patients and their carers.

Mastery of theoretical knowledge

Theoretical knowledge is continually changing, as more research into complementary therapies is being published. Research can contribute to the development of a therapist's knowledge and practice as new evidence-based innovations are investigated, evaluated and implemented. Irvine (1997) argues that mastery has a high degree of technical knowledge and skill, unsupervised responsibility in the work and a strong sense of accountability, personal self-discipline and rigour. However, it could be argued that mastery is not a static state but a process through careful investigation, curiosity about one's work and willingness to be open and reflective. There can be a downside to masterful practice, in that the authority engendered might disempower those who are served by the profession (Illich 1977). For therapists working with people with cancer, an authoritarian approach would be unhelpful. The work seeks to connect with others, and explores through the therapeutic use of touch the patient's needs in terms of comfort and support. The mechanisms of action for massage and bodywork may never be fully understood. This mystery itself is essential to remaining open and curious about the work. It can also be argued that taking a more objective and investigative view through research may make therapists more effective practitioners (Lewith 2004). It is important for therapists to continually develop their knowledge and skills so that they can offer the most effective service to patients and carers.

Problem solving/self-enhancement

One of the challenges facing complementary therapies is that, realistically, the benefits are largely viewed as supportive and not curative (House of Lords 2000). Key questions raised by the House of Lords Report were: Is the therapy safe in practice? Does it provide the benefits claimed? Is it cost effective compared to other tried and tested interventions?

At a personal level, therapists need to reflect on their own performance, develop new insights and co-operate in policy and practical matters (Hoyle & John 1995) (see Chapter 1). The education and regulation of massage therapists has been the focus of much criticism (Foundation for Integrated Medicine (FIM) 1997). It could be argued that poorly prepared therapists who do not pursue continuing education hold back professional development of complementary therapies. There has been a tradition in education of learning by transmission of knowledge and acquisition of skills from the teacher(s). Learning can be facilitated by mentors and involve active processes such as reflective practice, problem solving and student-led seminars and workshops.

Supervision is one approach which helps therapists to become confident and able to deal with problems, and to become more resourceful and autonomous in their work. In this context, supervision is understood to be central to the process of learning, expansion of the scope of practice, and a means of encouraging assessment, analytical and reflective skills (Hawkins & Shohet 1989, Tavares 2003). While supervision is also considered to be an effective risk management tool (Tingle 1995), for it to be welcomed and effective, it must also be viewed as useful, safe and appropriate to the supervisee's practice (Mackereth 2000). A useful skill for therapists is reflective practice so they can learn from incidents which have occurred. Other useful skills therapists could develop through supervision are contracting, establishing boundaries, time management and working with a person-centred approach.

However, there is no statutory requirement for supervision. The challenge to introduce this supportive and professional development strategy demands flexible models that meet local needs, training and education, and the building of relationships which are helpful for sustaining and developing practice. Examples of the different ways in which supervision has been developed for complementary therapists in palliative care settings are given in Box 4.3.

Continuing education is judged to be a necessary process to ensure safe and continual improvement of practice and a hallmark of professional self-regulation (Budd & Mills 2000). There are many ways to do this (see Box 4.4), but perhaps the most important factor is an individual's motivation for the activity. Other factors for consideration include time, funding, and suitable availability of cancer-specific educational opportunities. Some professional organisations make ongoing personal development a condition of continuing membership and members are expected to prove that the mandatory number

---

Box 4.3
Examples of supervision methods

- One supervisor to one supervisee.
- One supervisor to a small group of supervisees – during work time or in the evening.
- Complementary therapy (CT) co-ordinator supervises own team.
- Non-management supervision, e.g. external supervisor, supervisor from another clinical specialty, CT co-ordinator from another centre, such as on a mutual exchange basis.
- List of supervisors from which the therapist can choose.
- Commitment to 4–6 weekly supervision.

Mackereth (2000), Tavares (2003).

Box 4.4
Examples of different ways professional development needs can be met

- Reflective practice, incorporating a structured review of events, responses and other options.
- Clinical supervision – contracted monthly individual or group sessions facilitated by an experienced practitioner.
- Mentoring – regular supportive contact with an experienced practitioner.
- Educational events – attendance at conferences, study days and workshops.
- Journal club – each member reports back on an article/chapter/educational events.
- Peer-support group – regular meetings to exchange treatments and share practice issues.
- Networking and communicating regularly with colleagues by post, telephone and email.
- Accessing information via Internet, libraries, association newsletters and professional journals.

of hours has been completed, for example 10–12 hours a year. This will usually need to be confirmed by verification and certification.

Creation of a subculture

As groups strive for 'professionalism' they usually form subcultures, where certain procedures, rules and language are used by a group of people. For example, there may be a need to form local groups of similarly qualified and like-minded therapists, to have annual conferences, to form committees and to have shared practices and codes of conduct. Concessions are given to members of the group and although outsiders are welcome, they may not receive the same privileges (e.g. discounts on fees). Some therapists may use words and concepts which may not be understood by others. This makes the meaning of some interactions exclusive to those that are 'in the know' (e.g. auric cleansing, flushing toxins and channelling of energy). Care must be taken to avoid a culture of exclusivity that risks disempowering service users and novice therapists.

LEADERSHIP THROUGH AWARENESS AND FACILITATION

This chapter has explored the characteristics of a profession alongside key elements that protect, ensure permission and support potent therapeutic work. As a therapist develops and gains confidence through experience and processes of self-enhancement, there is a great potential for the emergence of effective role models and leaders in the provision of massage and bodywork in cancer care settings. Figure 4.1 summarises key concepts from this chapter and illustrates facilitative activities that can enable therapists to maximise their skills, knowledge and expertise in this area. Although not discussed in this chapter, therapists may also be helped by the support of social and family structures alongside education and supervision to achieve personal and pro-

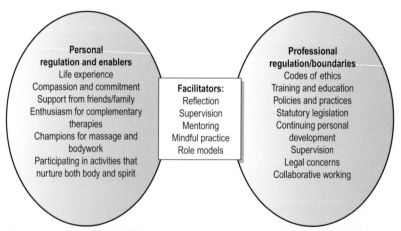

Figure 4.1   Model for facilitating professional and potent practice.

fessional goals. It is also possible that therapists can be helped to develop and flourish in their role by the support of champions (e.g. medical, nursing, managerial colleagues, service users and carers) who encourage, promote and even help obtain funding for the provision of massage and bodywork (Mackereth & Stringer 2005).

The establishment of teams of therapists in cancer care settings has led to the development of a co-ordinator's role (Tavares 2003). In time, these individuals with further development and experience will facilitate others through being effective role models, and mentoring and sharing their expertise. Therapists in cancer care, mindful of the vulnerability of patients and the journey, are working at the edge of practice, finding creative, safe and innovative methods and approaches to delivering treatments. Johns (2004) in exploring the concept of mindful practice with patients in palliative care settings, suggests it can also be 'the conscious dwelling with other care practitioners towards harmonising the caring effort and to grow through the care experience' (p. 19). Leadership can be in the everyday moment of working, by staying in awareness, and having a heartfelt willingness to be open and share with others what has been learnt and has yet to be learnt.

A major challenge for health professionals and complementary therapists alike is to maintain and develop practice and high-quality service. It is important to find ways of avoiding becoming exhausted and overwhelmed by the challenges and losses that can occur when working in cancer care (Lyckholm 2001). There are many ways to avoid burnout including having regular support and supervision and participating in activities that nurture the body and spirit. For some, this can involve a regular spiritual practice (e.g. meditation, prayer), receiving massage, eating healthily and participating in physical activities (e.g. swimming, dancing). In recognising that being a therapist can be a healing process in itself, Mackereth (1998, p. 25) advocates that to engage therapeutically and safely, and with the emphasis on 'being' rather than 'doing', it requires:

> an open heart, and willingness to journey with others, but to acknowledge that I have my own needs and issues for which I require support. I believe healing can take place if I can be with others and be myself in a way that defines our boundaries and helps create sacred space for healing.

SUMMARY

This chapter has explored the characteristics of professional working in the context of the '3 Ps' – protection, permission and potency. It is likely that professional and potent practice leads to greater job satisfaction and helps to avoid burnout, as well as continually motivating therapists to develop both personally and professionally. Recommendations made in Box 4.5 are to support therapists in their work and professional development. The potential

---

Box 4.5
Recommendations for potent and professional practice

- Therapists need to be adaptable, and be able to acknowledge their boundaries in terms of knowledge and skills to themselves and others.
- Reflective practice/supervision should be ongoing to help therapists develop strengths and to explore ways of resolving challenges.
- Therapists need to be aware of their individual and personal need for support, ongoing self-enhancement and activities that nurture the body and spirit.
- Inherent in an emerging profession is the need for a culture of facilitation to flourish that enables others to grow and develop.
- Professionals need to work within an ethical framework, mindful of their duty of care, to respect a patient's autonomy and acknowledging their own limitations.
- Innovations in care need champions and supporters. These can be friends, colleagues, service users and volunteers.
- Care must be taken to ensure that in developing professionally, therapists do not become inward looking or static (e.g. use exclusive language), but remain open and curious about their work.
- Recognition that therapists in cancer care settings are working at the edge of practice, finding creative, safe and innovative methods of working.
- Mindful practice can assist in being present as a therapist bringing comfort and support through touch, as well as contributing to the wider care environment.

---

of potent practice is not only to enrich the service today, but also to influence the future provision of integrated and person-centred massage and bodywork therapy in cancer care.

REFERENCES

Beauchamp TL, Childress JF 1994 Principles of biomedical ethics, 4th edn. Oxford University Press, Oxford

Budd S, Mills S 2000 Regulatory prospects for complementary and alternative medicine: information pack. Centre for Complementary Health Studies University of Exeter on behalf of the Department of Health

Cohen MH 2003 Regulation, religious experience, and epilepsy: a lens on complementary therapies. Epilepsy and Behaviour 4:602–606

Crossman P 1966 Permission and protection. Transactional Analysis Bulletin 5(19):152–154

Daniel R 2001 Holistic approaches to cancer: general principles and the assessment of the patient. In: Barraclough J (ed) Integrated cancer care, holistic, complementary and creative approaches. Oxford University Press, Oxford

Dimond B 1995 Legal issues – complementary therapies and the nurse. Complementary Therapies in Nursing and Midwifery 1:21–23

Foundation for Integrated Medicine 1997 Integrated healthcare: a way forward for the next five years? Foundation for Integrated Medicine, London

Hawkins P, Shohet R 1989 Supervision in the helping professions. Open University Press, Buckingham

House of Lords Select Committee on Science and Technology 2000 Complementary and alternative medicine. HL Paper 123. House of Lords, London

Hoyle E, John PD 1995 Professional knowledge and professional practice. Cassell, London

Houle CO 1980 Continuing learning in the professions. Jossey-Bass, San Francisco

Illich I 1977 The disabling professions. Martin Boyers, London

Irvine DH 1997 The performance of doctors. professionalism and regulation in a changing world. BMJ 314:540–542

Johns C 2004 Being mindful, easing suffering. Jessica Kingsley, London

Kendrick K 1999 Challenging power, autonomy and politics in complementary therapies; a contentious view. Complementary Therapies in Nursing and Midwifery 5:77–81

Kohn M 1999 Complementary therapies in cancer: abridged report of a study produced for Macmillan Cancer Relief. Macmillan Cancer Relief, London

Lewith G 2004 Can practitioners be researchers? Complementary Therapies in Medicine 12(1):2–5

Lewith GT, Bromfield J, Prescott P 2002 Complementary cancer care in Southampton: a survey of staff and patients. Complementary Therapies in Medicine 10:100–106

Lyckholm L 2001 Dealing with stress, burnout, and grief in the practice of oncology. The Lancet Oncology 2(12):750–755

Mackereth PA 1998 Body, relationship and sacred space. Complementary Therapies in Nursing and Midwifery 4:125–127

Mackereth P 2000 Clinical supervision and complementary therapies. In: Rankin-Box D (ed) Nurses' handbook of complementary therapies. Churchill Livingstone, London

Mackereth P, O'Hara C 2002 Appreciating preparatory and continuing education. In: Mackereth P, Tiran D (eds) Clinical reflexology: a guide for health professionals. Churchill Livingstone, Edinburgh

Mackereth PA, Stringer J 2005 CAM and cancer care: champions for integration. Complementary Therapies in Clinical Practice 11(1):45–47

Rankin-Box D 1997 Therapies in practice: a survey assessing nurses' use of complementary therapies. Complementary Therapies in Nursing and Midwifery 3:92–99

Roberts D, McNulty A, Caress A 2005 Current issues in the delivery of complementary therapies in cancer care. Policy, perceptions and expectations: an overview. European Journal of Oncology Nursing 9(2):115–123

Stone J 2002 An ethical framework for complementary and alternative therapies. Routledge, London

Tavares M 2003 National guidelines for the use of complementary therapies in supportive and palliative care. The Prince's Foundation for Integrated Health, National Council for Hospice and Specialist Palliative Care Services, London

Tingle J 1990 Patient consent: the issues. Nursing Standard 5(9):52–54

Tiran D 1996 The use of complementary therapies in midwifery practice: a focus on reflexology. Complementary Therapies in Nursing and Midwifery 2:32–37

Vollmer H, Mills D 1966 Editor's introduction to professionalization, v–ix. Prentice-Hall, Englewood Cliffs, NJ

White P 1998 Potential problems of integrating complementary therapies into cancer care. Radiography 4:269–278

Wilkinson J, Peters D, Donaldson J 2004 Report. Clinical governance for complementary and alternative medicine (CAM) in primary care. University of Westminster, London

Wilkinson S 2002 Complementary therapies – patient demand. International Journal of Palliative Nursing 8(10):468

FURTHER READING

House of Lords Select Committee on Science and Technology 2000 Complementary and alternative medicine. HL Paper 123. House of Lords, London

Hunter M, Struve J 1998 The ethical use of touch in psychotherapy. Sage Publications, London

Molassiotis A, Cawthorn A, Mackereth P 2006 Complementary and alternative therapies in cancer care. In: Kearney N, Richardson A (eds) Nursing patients with cancer: principles and practice. Elsevier, London

USEFUL ADDRESSES

The Prince's Foundation for Integrated Health
33–41 Dallington Street
London EC1V 0BB
UK
Tel: 020 3119 3100
Fax: 020 3119 3101
E-mail: info@fih.org.uk

Linda Orrett
Integrated Therapies Training Unit
c/o The Rehabilitation Unit
Christie Hospital NHS Trust
Wilmslow Road
Manchester M20 4BX
Tel: 0161 446 8236

Working with the denied body

5

Anne Cawthorn

Abstract

This chapter addresses some of the issues arising for both patients and therapists when denial is used as a coping mechanism. Relevant literature is introduced from the field of psycho-oncology in relation to working with denial. The main focus is on how therapists can utilise a therapeutic model to integrate complementary and alternative medicine (CAM) therapies into cancer care in a way that will safely facilitate the patient's adjustment. This is explored through the use of case studies from the author's experience; the author works jointly with massage therapists to help patients to adjust and heal during their cancer journey.

KEYWORDS

denial, coping, touch, Chiron myth, therapeutic relationship, models

INTRODUCTION

When individuals are diagnosed as having cancer they may choose to cope by dealing with one problem at a time, using partial or total denial as a form of defence. Denial was described by Freud (1961) as the refusal to acknowledge the existence of a real situation or the feelings associated with it. In many cases denial operates as a healthy mechanism and protects a person from the immediate shock of reality. Davidhizar and Giger (1998) suggest that 'normally denial diminishes and the person begins to face and accept the harsh reality of what has been blocked out' (p. 44). Denial is also seen as a defence mechanism, which applies in relation to coping, and has an important role in protecting against unbearable anxiety (Wells 2000). Lazarus and Folkman (1984) define coping theory as the ability of an individual to manage internal and external demands, which are appraised as taxing or exceeding their personal resources.

A therapist who can work with patients to help them identify and work through the problems associated with their diagnosis and prognosis can be invaluable. This requires helping the patient to be aware of the purpose of defences resulting from old patterns of thinking, feeling and behaving and the accompanying bodily sensations (Erskine et al 1999). When working with denial the therapist needs to take care to assess the purpose and strength of denial. Maguire (1995) reminds us that these coping mechanisms serve a purpose and should only be challenged when the therapist has assessed that it is in the patient's best interest. However, Erskine et al (1999) remind us that defences are costly as they not only bar an individual from contact and growth, but they also take energy to maintain. Therapists need to be aware that a patient's denial might be adding to the burden of fatigue associated with both the illness and cancer treatments (Dougherty & Bailey 2001).

THE CHIRON MYTH

Kearney (1997) suggests that the Chiron myth can serve as a useful model for the stages that patients may experience from denial through to acceptance. Case study 5.1 illustrates the use of the Chiron myth in a therapeutic context. Each stage is explained by reference to the patient's progress through the stages. Chiron was a mythical character, half horse, half human, and half mortal, half immortal. Chiron thought that he was immortal until an arrow wounded his knee. This left him with an agonising and unhealable wound. Chiron's wound became symbolic and meaningful in helping his understanding and healing work with the suffering of others.

Case study 5.1
The five stages of the Chiron myth (Kearney 1997)

Norma, a 41-year-old woman, was diagnosed as having ovarian cancer. This diagnosis left her feeling mortally wounded and she was having difficulty adjusting to the situation. Norma had been brought up in a family that discounted any reference to her pain, hunger, etc. As a consequence she discounted her symptoms, which were telling her to rest and take care of herself. Therapy involved helping Norma to re-learn the ability to listen to her body, giving her permission that it was okay to do so.

STAGE 1: THE WOUNDING

Chiron was wounded by an arrow and for Norma the wound was the diagnosis of a life-threatening illness. Kearney (1997) suggests that this wounding links with earlier woundings. For Chiron it was being abandoned by his parents, whereas for Norma it was associated with her abusive upbringing. Kearney suggests that to facilitate adjustment, therapists need to offer support with problems relating to earlier issues as well as current ones.

STAGE 2: THE STRUGGLE

For Chiron this entailed a desperate search to find a cure. For Norma, the struggle was maintaining a 'workaholic' existence. Norma totally denied what she was doing to her body. Her surgical wound was failing to heal, as was her ability to emotionally and physical cope with the situation. Working with Norma through this stage entailed developing a relationship, offering emotional support and physical contact through the use of massage and reflexology.

STAGE 3: THE CHOICE

The choice for Chiron entailed moving from the heroic stance to making decisions about the future. Kearney (1997) describes this as a paradigm shift to uncharted territories. The problem/situation remains, but one's perception of it can change. As Norma was still left with small tumours in her abdomen, the therapist used imagery and dream work to help her to alter the way she perceived these. She learned to accommodate them and make friends with them, thereby adjusting to their presence.

STAGE 4: THE DESCENT

The descent involves stepping beyond the familiar into the world of the unconscious. Chiron died and went into the underworld. Norma went through the stages of grieving for her old life and the losses the illness had forced upon her. This was a painful stage, but necessary in working towards adjustment. During this time, psychotherapy helped her to work through the problems associated with the initial wounding and her current illness.

STAGE 5: THE RETURN

Chiron eventually returned to his village, but he was never the same again. Norma changed her workaholic existence to find a complete career change. This was achieved through therapy, which encouraged Norma to confront her discounts and to become aware of her needs. One particularly poignant session involved the use of dreams. Norma described a dream in which she saw a china doll that had been badly damaged. In her dream, Norma did not think that it could be mended, it was so badly damaged. Through the use of imagery, Norma returned the doll to its original intact state. When this happened Norma realised that the doll symbolised her old wounds and the imagery facilitated healing of her past experience. The image of her as a whole intact person represented adjustment, and over time Norma made the necessary changes in her life to make this possible.

The therapist needs to understand and respect the patient's reasons for adopting denial so that therapeutic approaches, which can result in healing and growth, may be adopted. The goal in helping patients to work with denial is for them to achieve adjustment. Brennan (2001) refers to the notion of adjustment as originating from the Darwinian theory of 'adaptation', whereby the species adapted to the dangers of the physical world. In the past this may have been by utilising the fight or flight mechanism to run away from predatory animals. Our modern day stressors are somewhat different and therefore our previous coping mechanisms of running away or withdrawing may not be of use when coping with cancer and its treatments (although the urge to do this may still be present).

WORKING WITHIN AN INTEGRATIVE MODEL

In order to support patients, therapists need to have a way of working which will help them to offer safe holistic care. This can include working within an integrative model that is complementary to the patient's medical care. When making an assessment it is essential that issues relating to denial are included. The therapist also needs to develop and maintain a high level of self-awareness throughout the emerging therapeutic relationship. This also includes body awareness during therapeutic encounters (for both the patient and the therapist). The Integrative Model of Holistic Care (IMHC) takes into account the medical system. (The model was first developed by Michael Kearney, a palliative care consultant, and has been integrated into the author's work as a CAM practitioner in the field of cancer care (Cawthorn & Mackereth 2005).) The IMHC involves a holistic approach where CAM therapies are offered alongside medical care. This allows a therapy to be safely offered in a way that bridges complementary and conventional care and includes working with the 'person', adapting a therapeutic intervention and creating a special space (see Figure 5.1).

UNDERTAKING A HOLISTIC ASSESSMENT

The psychotherapist works in partnership with the client so that all aspects in relation to denial are addressed. Apart from eliciting patient concerns, psychological assessment should include any denial and/or discounting and the impact on the patient's coping mechanisms. The psychotherapist needs to ascertain the extent of the denial, whether it is complete or partial, or whether there is a window in the denial, through which, if appropriate, it could be challenged. The therapist needs to assess what purpose the denial serves and whether it is having a negative effect on the patient and/or on others.

An important area in working with denial is assessing the patient's coping mechanisms. Studies into patients' individual adjustment styles have led many workers in the field of oncology to question how denial impacts on the client's ability to adjust. Barraclough (1999) refers to psychodynamic models of adaptation undertaken by Freud (1856–1939) to explain adjustment. The theory

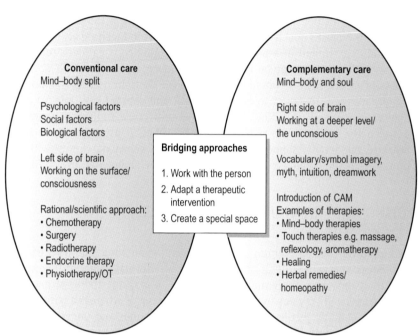

Figure 5.1   The Integrative Model of Holistic Care (Kearney 2000, adapted by Cawthorn 2004). OT, occupational therapy; CAM, complementary and alternative medicine.

asserts that adjustment is based on the belief that early developmental experiences and relationships, combined with instinctive drives, continue to influence a person's feelings and behaviour throughout life. So when a patient is faced with the loss of control and threat of dependence imposed by cancer, attempts to regain control are made unconsciously through enhancing defences learned in childhood. Defences can include: denial, projection, displacement, sublimation, regression, intellectualisation and conversion (Barraclough 1999). A study by Greer et al (1979) into adjustment styles of women with breast cancer (n = 69) has been a template for many other studies. Prior to surgery the women were psychologically assessed for depression and social adjustment. Adjustment styles were identified and later clarified by Moorey and Greer (2002) as: fatalism (stoical acceptance), positive avoidance (denial), helpless/hopeless fighting spirit, and anxious preoccupation.

It is important for any therapist to remember that when faced with a stressful situation patients usually adopt the preferred coping style that often made them feel secure when younger. This does not necessarily mean that it is currently helping the situation, but it may feel familiar. For example someone with fighting spirit to discount the extent and significance of his pain would be normal. The opposite may be the case for someone for whom anxious preoccupation is the favoured coping style. Patients can move between these coping styles as they are not rigid. If positive avoidance is the preferred style, then the therapist's goal is to work with the patient to facilitate acknowledgement and adjustment of a problem. In clinical practice, a patient's refusal of a massage treatment may be an unhelpful avoidance. She may still want the massage yet she says, 'It would be too much for me right now'. It is important for the massage therapist to accept her 'no' and support her right to make choices in the here and now. A psychotherapist could support a patient to examine the hesitation to receive touch therapies. A psychotherapist could rehearse the activity supporting her responses in achieving control with the proviso that she could ask for the treatment to be stopped at any point.

DEVELOPING AND MAINTAINING A HIGH LEVEL OF SELF-AWARENESS

It is important for all therapists to develop and maintain a high level of self-awareness. This allows therapists to be aware of information about themselves that may impact on the patient. For example, a massage therapist may feel comfortable and very positive about receiving massage whereas a patient who views his body as 'letting him down' may feel anxious and uncertain about physical touch. Self-awareness for the therapist comes about through personal reflection, individual, group or peer supervision and personal therapy. When reflecting on relationships and work with patients, it is essential to assess if the therapist is fully aware of personal thoughts, feelings, behaviours and bodily sensations when working with patients with cancer. Patients are coping with both the diagnosis of cancer and subsequent treatments, and are also coming to terms with their own mortality. It is important to note that denial can occur not only for the patients and carers but also for therapists. Therapists may need to address whether denial is present for them through supervision. Areas to consider for them may be around the diagnosis, treatment and threat to mortality. Certain patients can raise a therapist's awareness of his own mortality, which might lead a therapist to discount certain responses. One response could be to blocking discussions about death and dying by changing the subject, as a way of maintaining personal defence mechanisms. For massage therapists who struggle with treating patients with cancer due to their own defence mechanisms and own transferential issues (see Chapter 6), appropriate training and support could be helpful when working through these issues. A therapist's reluctance to massaging patients with cancer may be linked to early experiences and fears informing their knowledge and feelings about the causes, treatment and outcomes of cancer.

THE EMERGING AND DEVELOPING THERAPEUTIC RELATIONSHIP

Any therapist needs to develop and maintain a therapeutic relationship which is essential when working with patients, but is especially important if discounting is evident. The primary task therefore of any therapist should be to initiate and develop the therapeutic contract. The need to form relationships is the essence of human functioning. As therapists, this is developed by attuning to the individual's needs using genuine contact and connectedness, which encourages awareness and disarms defences. The therapeutic relationship involves the coming together of two separate people, each with their own thoughts, feelings, behaviours and bodily sensations. How therapists work with patients depends on the therapies in which they are competent and are able to offer. The extent to which the relationship develops depends upon how far the therapist has travelled on their personal journey of self-development. Therapists will only be able to take the patient as far as they have travelled within the appropriate boundaries of practice. However, patients may move forward in their processes, including working through denial and discounting through other interventions, such as massage or indeed with the support of friends and family. For some people the journey with cancer is complex and overwhelming, requiring the expertise of appropriately qualified psychotherapists and counsellors.

Developing the therapeutic relationship is like a dance. Some patients will immediately be in step, whereas others will need extra help from the therapist to pay attention to and be mindful of the steps they take. Patients who are using defence mechanisms as a way of coping may not be fully engaged in the dance. In fact, some may actively be 'sitting this one out'. The therapist's skill is in inviting them on to the dance floor, guiding and showing them that they can trust in the relationship. With time and patience, they may allow the therapist into their worlds and in turn help them learn a new empowering, carefree, contactful dance. Therapists and patients will know when this has been achieved as each will be fully aware of genuine thoughts, feelings, behaviours and bodily sensations. This can be a real 'Aha' moment of realisation and satisfaction. Just as the dance engaged in may be different within each session, so the dynamics of the relationship can alter from session to session.

Dynamics of the Emergent Relationship Model

The author has observed that patients in a cancer care setting may come for a first therapy session presenting one of five emergent relationships (see Box 5.1). A patient may remain in this relationship throughout the session. For example, a patient can arrive in the **now** relationship, but as the therapy progresses, existential issues emerge, leading the therapist to move into working with the **soulful** relationship. Another example is where the patient presents in the **wanting** relationship, but as a result of an additional intervention such as massage, his needs are met. By the end of the therapy session the patient is in the **now** relationship. This shift may happen when the therapist's nurturing touch reminds patients of their mother's touch, although the mother may no longer be available to offer nurturing. Patients may or may not recognise that they needed this prior to receiving a massage. However, what commonly happens is that skilled therapists will be able to work in any of the five relationships and change their way of working to match, or

> ### Box 5.1
> ### The Emergent Relationship Model
>
> - The **now** relationship – working as partners in an adult-to-adult relationship.
> - The **wanting** relationship – where the therapist is aware that the client is vulnerable or needy, i.e. the therapist may be aware that they are not working as adult to adult, but like a nurturing parent to child.
> - The **evoked** relationship – involves transference and counter-transference. Somatised feelings are utilised in the work.
> - The **soulful** relationship – often clients who are coming to terms with a life-threatening or life-limiting illness begin to consider their own mortality.
> - The **uncovered** relationship – the therapist is either presented with, or deliberately chooses to use, information gained from the patient's subconscious.

complement that of the patients. This model will now be examined in relation to psychotherapy and massage practice.

The Emergent Relationship Model in practice

First, the **now** relationship means that the patient and therapist partnership is an adult-to-adult relationship which includes thoughts, feelings, behaviours and bodily sensations, congruent to the present situation. If denial is used as a coping mechanism it is more likely to be because it is out of the client's or therapist's awareness, or as a planned strategy for dealing with a situation that is difficult to cope with. For example, the patient may know, on one level, that he has a poor prognosis. However, he may be coping by choosing not to focus on it, while trying to make the most of the limited time available. In massage, the therapist needs to honour this use of denial when treating patients, avoiding the temptation to lead to conversations that may be regretted after leaving the intimate environment of a therapy room. Creating a special and safe space respects the **now** needs of a patient. It should not be the agenda of a therapist to move the patient on to where he does not want to go at present.

The **wanting** relationship is where the therapist is aware that the client is vulnerable or needy. One way of assessing if the therapist is working in this domain is to be aware of the dynamics of the relationship. On reflection, the therapist may be aware that she is offering a nurturing parental relationship as the client may have regressed to exhibiting thoughts, feelings and behaviours more akin to child ego states. Berne (1972) recommends that in this situation the therapist makes friends with the 'child' in order that they will become more grounded and eventually be able to use more of their adult resources. The patient in a child state may seek comfort from the therapist, clinging to the relationship and become anxious if the massage therapist is on holiday. People who are vulnerable need support at that particular time. The massage therapist could suggest other support available during their absence. For example the patient could be introduced to a trusted colleague who works in a similar way. The patient makes the choice to arrange an appointment. Working in this way can be perceived as the therapist becoming a companion to the patient. The poem 'Footprints' (Fishback Powers 1993) describes what being a companion entails: 'A true companion will be strong enough to accompany them, staying in step'. At times the following may also apply: 'During your trials and testings, when you saw one set of footprints, it was then that I carried you' (p. 63). A competent therapist will be able to evaluate whether their role as companion required two sets of footprints or whether, on occasions only one set was present, which was when the patient was vulnerable or needy.

The **evoked** relationship involves the therapist bringing transferential and counter-transferential material (see Chapter 6), which can emerge and complicate the therapeutic work. Clinical supervision affords therapists a useful format to clarify what the issues relate to. For example, if a therapist is feeling nauseous and 'churned up' when working with an anxious patient, she may wish to consider what information this provides about herself. Alternatively, the information that has been picked up via the transference can be useful to the work with a patient. For example, if a massage therapist considers that a churning feeling, while working patients' feet, might be valuable information in relation to the patient's bodily sensations, she may wish to share this as a way of giving the patient more information about what is happening. The best way to do this is to come from a place of curious enquiry. The therapist could start by saying what was experienced and then ask if it relates to the patient. In this way it allows the patient to acknowledge it or deny it, thereby keeping the relationship intact. So when the feet were being massaged the patient might have been feeling emotional about the quality of attention being given. A patient could say that it reminded them of the loving touch given by their mother when the patient was a child. The massage therapist could acknowledge the power of the experience, while a psychotherapist may encourage patients to examine their feelings more.

The **soulful** relationship is where the patient is beginning to consider the existential implications of being diagnosed with a life-threatening or life-limiting illness. Cancer can affect many aspects of a patient's life, not least the emotional, spiritual and social dimensions. Often patients are forced prematurely into acknowledging their own mortality, which can leave them isolated, vulnerable and doubting previous coping strategies. Experienced mind–body therapists can play an important role in reducing the existential anxiety by accompanying them on their journey, working through their losses and acknowledging their isolation and vulnerability. In massage a patient may drift into a deeply relaxed state where questions emerge about the meaning of the illness and thoughts of a spiritual nature. Again the massage therapist can acknowledge these as important and transforming, whereas a psychotherapist would encourage the patient to examine these thoughts more closely in relationship to their illness and future.

The **uncovered** relationship is where the therapist negotiates to work with the patient utilising the unconscious aspects of the brain in order to access information which may not be readily available when using the left logic side. The therapist needs to be trained in this type of work and receive ongoing supervision. Care should always taken to ensure that the client is in agreement to work in this way, and also that there are no underlying psychiatric problems which could contraindicate this work. An example of working with the **uncovered** relationship is given in Case study 5.2.

Case study 5.2

Belinda, aged 24, had successfully received treatment for thyroid cancer. She had a needle phobia and often ran out of the waiting area prior to blood tests. Having undertaken a phobia cure with Belinda, the therapist was still considering that the problem was more complex. However, the answer came in the use of imagery as information was accessed from her unconscious. Once relaxed, the therapist asked Belinda to look at her arms and describe what she saw. To her amazement, the skin covering the inside of her arms appeared extremely thin, leaving her veins exposed and vulnerable. (Belinda decided her response to blood tests was to protect her arms.) Belinda said 'Yes' when asked if she wanted them to look normal again. The therapist encouraged her to choose a colour of fluid which she would find healing. She chose turquoise and imagined this magic fluid washing over her arms and healing the skin. After a while both arms returned to normal, first the right and then the left. On opening her eyes, she was amazed at what she had seen, initially the fragility of her arms and then later how they changed after the healing imagery. Subsequently, Belinda reported that she was able to stay and have her blood tests with no further problems.

Case study 5.3 demonstrates an example of where a patient who was initially in the **wanting** relationship moved into the **soulful** relationship when discussing dying. The dream work involved was in the **uncovered** relationship, while there was an acknowledgement that much of the work focused on transferential issues from the **evoked** relationship. As a result of combined use of therapy, the patient began to work much more in the **now** relationship.

Case study 5.3

Julie, aged 33, was receiving palliative chemotherapy for advanced ovarian disease. Arriving at the initial session on the ward, the therapist witnessed Julie experiencing a panic attack. On questioning, Julie disclosed that she was extremely anxious about the future and stated that she was frightened of dying. Observing her, it was obvious that she was using regression as a defence mechanism. Julie seemed very young, afraid to get out of bed, or to be left alone. In the first session, the therapist elicited her existential fears by creating a special space in which to contain her anxieties. On the second visit Julie had just woken up from a frightening dream. The therapists worked with her to facilitate a satisfactory ending to the dream, as it seemed symbolic of the helpless position in which she found herself.

Reflecting on the first visit, the therapist had suggested that she could act as a companion; only one set of footprints were visualised with the therapist carrying her. However, following the second session, there were two sets of footprints as Julie connected with her adult resources and began participating in rehabilitation activities. Later on, the therapists helped Julie to learn how to manage her anxiety and panic attacks, and to accept and enjoy massage treatments from the team.

BRINGING THE BODY INTO THE THERAPEUTIC ENCOUNTER

The psychotherapist when working in cancer care needs to consider bringing the body into the therapeutic encounter. For the massage therapist this is the focus from the start, but methods of engagement and exploration are different. Both need to bring their own thoughts, feelings, behaviours and bodily sensations into their reflections when working with patients to inform the contact and connection. The information gained should only be shared if it is considered to be appropriate; for example, in psychotherapy, if it will help to move the relationship forward. An example of where it is useful in massage is when areas of tension are palpated and the therapist brings it to the attention of the client – How does this muscle feel? Bringing the body into the therapeutic encounter can be undertaken in three ways: through the experience and responses to touch and bodywork interventions, by an exploration of embodiment in talk, and through imagery, visualisation and hypnotherapy exploring the unconscious.

Touch and bodywork

Autton (1989) reminds us how important the role of touch plays in our survival and security. It is a fundamental experience for exploring the world, finding sources of nourishment, seeking reassurance and contact with caregivers who provide protection and comfort (Field 2001), without which infants can fail to thrive and develop (Montagu 1986). The therapeutic use of touch therapies, such as massage, can be both an intentional and intuitive act. The individual-ised use of massage, as opposed to simply performing techniques, can be described as combining intentional and intuitive touch to meet and work with the person in the moment (Mackereth 2000). An example is described in Case study 5.4.

Case study 5.4

Sonia, aged 47, had undergone extensive surgery to the head and neck for oral cancer. This had left her with numerous scars and difficulty talking. By massag-ing the face, neck and chest the massage therapist was intentionally communi-cating her acceptance of her altered body image. The impact of the massage was to begin facilitating the adjustment process to her body image. The therapist intuitively sensed that Sonia was in need of touch as she 'soaked up' the rhythmic strokes of the massage in a way that a dry leaf soaks up moisture. The amount of touch she had received had been limited as her husband had recently died and her children were being cared for in her own country. Sonia reported needing the touch to help keep her safe and secure.

Touch therapies can play an important part in helping a patient to acknowl-edge the physical effects of stress and anxiety. Often a highly stressed patient will say after a massage: 'I did not realise how much tension I was holding in my shoulders'. There may be many reasons for a patient not addressing the physical symptoms of stress and anxiety, aside from denying the body. These can include being unable to find time for a therapy, or not feeling comfortable or confident in asking for help. For men, researchers have reported that seeking support can be like 'entering the unknown' (Miller 2003, p. 16). It is also possible that a patient may not feel she deserves help, and even being so disconnected from the body that awareness can only be achieved from the physical experience and acknowledgement of relaxation when receiving touch and massage. The power of touch to reveal previously contained and dis-embodied stress can be extremely profound. This cathartic release of deep emotions from touch interventions has been well documented in massage and bodywork literature (Mackereth 1999, Vickers 1996). The therapist's response to emotional release must be patient led, for example, simply stopping the massage and 'being with' the person may suffice. Patients may wish to explore feelings and thoughts in further work with a counsellor or psychotherapist (see recommendations in Box 5.2).

It is not uncommon for massage and bodywork therapists to report having tuned into and even felt a patient's emotional state just before it surfaces,

Box 5.2
Recommendations for therapists working with the 'denied body'

- Understanding the role of denial for people diagnosed with cancer.
- Being aware of a patient's past experience which might influence response and adjustment to cancer.
- Understanding the psychotherapeutic approaches to working with patients in cancer care.
- Examining the massage therapist's own concerns about working with people living and dying with cancer.
- Clarifying motivations for working in the field of cancer care.
- Developing awareness of somatic responses of both therapist and patient.
- Engaging in reflective practice and supervision to maintain and develop skills and safe practice.
- Appreciating and acknowledging boundaries of practice, and where appropriate guiding patients, with their permission, to seek psychotherapy or counselling.

which Eiden (2002) describes as a 'resonance' with a patient's own internal processes. Osteopath and psychotherapist Robert Shaw (2003) recommends that therapists actively bring the somatic phenomena that they feel while working in the therapeutic encounter to their own consciousness. Shaw (2003) believes that 'the therapist's body is an actively present agent and highly tuned to receiving information' (p. 24). If therapists are able to tune in to what they are experiencing and decide whether the sensations are those of the therapist or the patient, then they have more information to offer when working with patients. A therapist's decision to disclose this knowledge to the patient will depend upon how well developed the relationship is and how open patients are to being in the relationship and talking about their body. If body awareness is central to the therapist's approach to the work then it should be made explicit in the information provided early in developing the therapeutic contract (see Chapter 4 for further discussion).

Including imagery and creative visualisation

Another approach to bringing the body into the therapeutic encounter is through the use of techniques which access the unconscious mind, the right side of the brain (see Figure 5.1). The use of imagery, visualisation and hypnotherapy is emerging as an important way of working with patients. An area in cancer care where guided imagery has developed is in the field of psychoneuroimmunology (PNI) research, where the connection between the immune system and imagery has been extensively studied (see Further reading). There is evidence that the mind (psychology), brain (neurology) and body's immune system (immunology) communicate with each other (Ader 1996,

Watkins 1997). The concept that every thought, idea and belief is part of the mind–body pathways raises interesting questions of their role in maintaining health and fighting disease. The potential for using these findings when directly working with patients using imagery is proving to be an exciting area. Various levels are used from simple relaxation and visualisation to the use of hypnotherapy including strategies to manage anxiety, phobia and panic. The use of imagery can have a powerful effect to bring 'hidden aspects' of the self into awareness, or as a method of positively changing an altered body image. An example is given in Case study 5.5. Imagery and visualisation can also be used in a touch and massage context to deepen relaxation and awareness (see Chapter 14). The therapist would need to be trained and supervised in these techniques and the work contracted for with the patient (see Chapter 16).

Case study 5.5

Wendy, aged 44, had undergone a radical hysterectomy for ovarian cancer. She was left feeling 'empty internally' and thought that her scar was much redder than the therapist observed it to be. With the use of imagery techniques Wendy was encouraged to look inside and to tell the therapist what she saw. Wendy was not surprised to see a hole in her abdomen. The therapists asked her if she wanted to fill this, which she did. Using an imagery technique by Leuner (1984) Wendy was encouraged to imagine that she was filling it up with 'magic fluid'. Wendy followed the therapist's suggestion and imagined the 'magic fluid' to be peach coloured. Directly following the imagery she stated that this technique had 'filled the hole' and that her scar was less inflamed. This changed body image allowed her to adjust to the changes following her surgery.

SUMMARY

This chapter has examined and explored psychotherapy and its relationship to massage and bodywork in practice. Case studies have been used to illuminate practical ways of working using therapeutic models and approaches. Recommendations have been made for massage and bodywork therapists to ensure safe and appropriate practice for working in the complex area of cancer care (see Box 5.2). This chapter has highlighted the advantages of massage therapists and psychotherapists working together and developing an understanding of each other's role, and the overlaps and potential in helping patients to integrate and heal the denied body.

REFERENCES

Ader R 1996 Historical perspectives on psychoneuroimmunology. In: Friedman H, Klein TW, Friedman AL (eds) Psychoneuroimmunology, stress and infection. CRC Press, Boca Raton, FL

Autton N 1989 Touch: an exploration. Darton, Longman & Todd, London

Barraclough J 1999 Cancer and emotion. A practical guide to psycho-oncology, 2nd edn. J Wiley & Sons, Chichester

Berne E 1972 What do you say after you say after you say hello? Bantam Books, New York

Brennan J 2001 Adjustment to cancer – coping or personal transition? Psycho-Oncology 10:1–18

Cawthorn A 2004 Using imagery and dreamwork. Poster presentation at the International Cancer Nursing Conference, 8–12 August, 2004, Sydney, Australia

Cawthorn A, Mackereth P 2005 Complementary and alternative therapies in rheumatology. In: Hill J (ed) Rheumatology nursing, 2nd edn. Whurr Publishers, London

Davidhizar R, Giger JN 1998 Patients' use of denial: coping with the unacceptable. Nursing Standard 12(43):44–46

Dougherty L, Bailey C 2001 Chemotherapy. In: Corner J, Bailey C (eds) Cancer care: care in context. Blackwell Science, Oxford

Eiden B 2002 Application of post-Reichian body psychotherapy: a Chiron perspective. In: Staunton T (ed) Body psychotherapy. Brunner-Routledge, Hove, East Sussex

Erskine RG, Moursund P, Trautmann RJ 1999 Beyond empathy. A therapy of contact-in-relationship. Edwards Brothers, Michigan

Field T 2001 Touch. The MIT Press, London

Freud S 1961 The ego and the id. Standard edition of the Complete Works of Freud, Vol XIX. Hogarth Press, London

Fishback Powers M 1993 Footprints. Marshall Pickering, London

Greer S, Morris T, Pettingale KW 1979 Psychological response to breast cancer: effect on outcome. The Lancet ii:785–787

Kearney M 1997 Mortally wounded stories of soul pain, death and healing. Touchstone, New York

Kearney M 2000 A place of healing. Working with suffering in living and dying. Oxford University Press, Oxford

Lazarus RS, Folkman S 1984 Stress appraisal and coping. Springer, New York

Leuner H 1984 Guided affective imagery – the basic course. Thieme-Stratton Inc, USA

Mackereth P 1999 An introduction to catharsis and the healing crisis in reflexology. Complementary Therapies in Nursing and Midwifery 5(3): 67–74

Mackereth P 2000 Tough places to be tender: contracting for happy or 'good enough' endings in therapeutic massage/bodywork? Complementary Therapies in Nursing and Midwifery 6(3):111–115

Maguire P 1995 Psychosocial interventions to reduce affective disorders. Cancer patients: research priorities. Psycho-Oncology 4:113–119

Millar A 2003 Men's experience of considering counselling: 'entering the unknown'. Counselling and Psychotherapy Research 3(1):16–24

Montagu A 1986 Touching: the human significance of skin. Harper & Row, New York

Moorey S, Greer S 2002 Psychological therapy for patients with cancer: a new approach, 2nd edn. Heinemann Medical Books, Oxford

Shaw R 2003 The embodied psychotherapist. Brunner-Routledge, Hove, East Sussex

Vickers A 1996 Massage and aromatherapy – a guide for health professionals. Chapman & Hall, London

Watkins A 1997 Mind–body medicine: a clinician's guide to psycho-neuroimmunology. Churchill Livingstone, New York

Wells M 2001 The impact of cancer. In: Corner J, Bailey C (eds) Cancer care: care in context. Blackwell Science, Oxford

FURTHER READING

Freeman LW 2001 Research on mind-body effects. In: Freeman LW, Lawlis GF (eds) Complementary and alternative medicine: a research-based approach. Mosby, London

Kübler-Ross E 1969 On death and dying. Tavistock, London

Molassiotis A, Cawthorn A, Mackereth P 2005 Complementary and alternative therapies. In: Kearney A, Richardson A (eds) Nursing patients with cancer. Principles and practice. Elsevier Science, London

Rubenfeld I 2000 The listening hand: how to combine bodywork and psycho-therapy to heal emotional pain. Piatkus, London

Tewes U 1999 Concepts in psychology. In: Schedlowski M, Tewes U (eds) Psychoneuroimmunology: an interdisciplinary introduction. Kluwer/Plenum Publishers, London

USEFUL ADDRESS

Anne Cawthorn
Nurse Psychotherapist
Psycho-Oncology Services
Holt House
Christie Hospital
Manchester M20 4BX
UK

6

Body psychotherapy in cancer care

Sue Hampton

Abstract

The author's training in body psychotherapy and transactional analysis influences the content of the chapter. The chapter describes body psychotherapy and its links with psychoneuroimmunology, three different approaches to body psychotherapy and an outline of the methods used. The tasks of both the therapist and the patient are included in a tabular form. The value of body psychotherapy to patients with cancer are explored. The chapter also includes feedback from a patient, a carer's case study and information about working with touch.

KEYWORDS

body psychotherapy, psychoneuroimmunology (PNI), trauma, Reich methods, transference and counter-transference

INTRODUCTION

The diagnosis of cancer can affect an individual in several ways. Elizabeth Kübler-Ross (1999) described the stages that people may go through as shock, numbness, denial, anger, acceptance and looking for a way forward. Not all workers in the field of supportive and palliative care agree with these stages. It has been argued that in reality they are too rigid and do not take account of individual life histories or coping strategies (Corr et al 1999, Kastenbaum 2004). A number of patients find that some emotions which surface are related to trauma, unpleasant memories and associated emotions from the past. These emotions may arise in addition to those which are concerned with coping with the illness, thus making life more distressing and healing more difficult. In the author's practice, it is mainly women who refer themselves to psychotherapy. Most of these women believe their cancers were linked to emotional causes or trauma, and they judged that psychotherapy could help attend to this aspect of their cancer care. These women have presented with a variety of issues, outlined in Box 6.1.

Box 6.1
Issues presented at a psychotherapy clinic for women with cancer

- History of divorce, separation or bereavement in childhood, or in the patient's own adult relationships.
- Alcohol, food and/or smoking, or overwork as a coping strategy, particularly when stressed, upset and/or lonely.
- Common perception of self as a caregiver and/or a good friend.
- Tendency to be self-effacing, but yet is over-controlling and over-functioning in relationships (this behaviour is due to an archaic belief that others are not responsible or capable).
- An underlying belief, 'I am only of value (can be important, can be safe, can belong, can be taken care of) if I take care of/or please others'.
- Has difficulty expressing emotion, such as fear, rage, grief and/or joy (parts of emotional self are suppressed).
- Unable or unwilling to express emotions such as resentment, rage, grief and/or joy (parts of themselves are kept hidden).
- Disruption of early attachment. For example, unavailable mother due to depression, distraction, disinterest or distress.

DEFINING BODY PSYCHOTHERAPY

Body psychotherapy is distinct from other bodywork therapies such as massage and reflexology because it also addresses the therapeutic relationship and its transferential aspects. Gentle massage, touch and holding may sometimes be used, but these techniques do not necessarily form the main part of the work as they do when used as a complementary therapy. The intent is one of transformation where the psychotherapist works alongside the body–mind processes of the patient. This body–mind connection is essential in enabling patients to reconnect with their 'authentic self'. The desired result is that a state of being is achieved where self-regulation, both psychological and physiological, can flourish. While other psychotherapeutic approaches recognise this reconnection as essential, body psychotherapy theory takes into account the complex interactions between body and mind. Candace Pert (1997, p. 274) in 'Molecules of Emotions' has succinctly identified how the mind has been split from the body in healthcare practice:

> Most psychologists treat the mind as disembodied, a phenomenon with little or no connection to the physical body. Conversely physicians treat the body with no regard to the mind or the emotions. But the body and mind are not separate, and we cannot treat one without the other . . . research has shown that the body can and must be healed through the mind and the mind can and must be healed through the body.

Carroll (2002), a body psychotherapist, suggested that working with the body helps a person 'to receive oneself'. Cameron (2002) describes this experience as 'proprioception', which can enable an individual to develop a body schema. This not only includes a physical image of self, but also an assessment of self-worth in relationship to others in the world/social context. The intention of any form of therapeutic touch and the attitude of the therapist may therefore contribute to informing and possibly revising the body schema.

WESTERN ROOTS OF BODY PSYCHOTHERAPY

In the 1920s, Wilhelm Reich, an Austrian psychiatrist, examined somatic (bodily) processes to broaden psychological theory and methodology. Reich (1973) developed a comprehensive theory linking character analysis, drive theory and body psychotherapy methodology. Although the root of his work was psychoanalytical, Reich's thinking moved away from that of Freud's as he opposed the body–mind split. Reich perceived thoughts and feelings as embodied phenomena, which could be processed directly through both bodily and verbal interventions. He argued therapeutic technique needed to include the physical domain to generate lasting change in psychic structure. In 1936, it was Reich's focus on the body, together with his political stance, that was the cause of his exclusion from the International Society of Psychoanalysis.

BODY PSYCHOTHERAPY DEVELOPMENT AND CURRENT THERAPIES

The great majority of current body psychotherapy is linked to Wilhelm Reich's work and his influence on the evolution of body psychotherapy is summarised in Appendix 6.1 at the end of the chapter. For completeness, many of the recognised body psychotherapy approaches currently available are detailed in Appendix 6.2.

PSYCHONEUROIMMUNOLOGY RESEARCH AND THE PATIENT WITH CANCER

Psychoneuroimmunology (PNI) studies the interrelationship between brain, behaviour and the immune system, and how the state of mind affects an individual's health. PNI research is providing evidence about the physiological connection between mind and body, and how this connection can be used to guide the body back to health. Dr Margo de Kooker (2001, p. 2) believes that:

> In the real world, what the field of PNI proves, is that what happens in our minds at the level of our perception, (and our emotional reaction to that perception), can have real effects on our physiology, (our physical response), and more specifically, our immune systems. This concept is not new, and ancient wisdom has always encouraged us to focus on maintaining a 'healthy' mind in order to maintain a healthy body. It is only now that we are able to prove and understand the connections.

What does PNI research mean to the patient living with cancer?

Patients who have hope and feel empowered, who are goal focused and informed, are more able to take charge of their situation and proactively work alongside their team of health professionals. Patients find that discussing the findings of PNI research can help to provide them with valuable information as they undergo treatment. Of particular value is the link between the body–mind and the immune system. The aim of a psychotherapist is to support patients so they can move into a position where they are in control of their own lives. The therapist can explain to patients that one of the ways in which they can use body psychotherapy is to develop a way of behaving and reacting to the condition that will support the health of their immune system. This encourages them to develop health-enhancing habits, which can be defined as 'immune power' traits (Dreher 1995). Such habits can shift the focus of attention away from illness towards living *more* fully. A treatment plan can be devised that works with the body–mind processes to support the health of the immune system and also avoids traumatising it further (for sources of information on PNI see Further reading).

Some aspects of deep change work can be very taxing and challenging. Three important areas are addressed and the methodology used works towards gentle and gradual change. First, the approach provides emotional and physical soothing, support and release. Second, by working with the patient's 'immune power' consciousness, the individual learns to support his or her immune system. Finally, most beneficial after medical treatment (because this can be the most psychologically challenging), patients are helped to dissolve historical patterns that they 'put in place' for protection, but which can also repress natural, healthy self-expression. Patients are empowered to develop a fuller sense of self and to create a life-enhancing existence. Patients with incurable cancer develop a greater sense of ease and acceptance during their last few months of life. Those patients in whom the cancer has been diagnosed and treated early enough can learn to contribute significantly (psychologically and behaviorally) to *possible* remission from the disease and prevention. Whatever the prognosis, patients can bring about profound changes to the way they live their lives.

INTEGRATION OF BODY PSYCHOTHERAPY IN PRACTICE

Nick Totton (2003) has identified three models of body psychotherapy, which are described below.

The Adjustment Model

This model has a corrective approach, which recognises the concept of body armouring (holding patterns), and supports the removal of these blocks to increase flow of energy. This model is useful for diagnosis, using character analysis and body mapping to identify visually and kinaesthetically the patient's repressed somatic trauma. The psychotherapist looks for the holding patterns, which are perceived to be expressions of the patient's unmet need or *interrupted impulse*. These diagnoses may be used to inform suggestions to patients about what they may need, or want to express, or validate.

The Trauma/Discharge Model

This model argues that the external trauma leads to a defensive freezing in the body. Healing occurs through emotional abreaction where repressed emotions are unblocked from rigid musculature so they can be fully experienced. However, with certain character structures, this way of working can lead to re-traumatising, particularly if the relationship between patient and therapist is insecure. The current trend is to work with a more gentle approach where patients are supported to manage their traumatic memory rather than reliving it. For the psychotherapist, this model can be used to give information about trauma and the effects it can have on the patient's physiological system. With a traumatised patient, and in the early stages of work with patients who have cancer, relaxation techniques and physical methods, such as gentle massage and breath work, can be used to help the patient induce the relaxation response. The relaxed state supports the functioning of the immune system.

The Process Model

In recent years, body therapies such as the Hakomi method (Kurtz 1990) have influenced another approach to body psychotherapy. The focus is on **how** patients communicate rather than the words being spoken. The language of the body can be more revealing than the spoken word. This model recognises that within the patient's body–mind, there is a story that is emerging, that wants to unfold. The role of the therapist is not to unblock the patient's armouring or trauma. Instead, the therapist maintains an open mind, and supports and follows the patient's body–mind processes through a therapeutic journey of exploration, experimentation and experience. Patients are encouraged to engage their thinking and awareness of physical sensations and to be curious about the stories that are held in their body; they are encouraged to move through interrupted impulses so that the story can unfold. In doing so, patients are able to connect to their embodied experiences and to gain access to their unconscious processes. In this way a patient can make meaning of their current condition and are able to address unmet need. This can be a particularly valuable method for patients with cancer, who require their therapist to stay alongside them, empathically and solidly, while undergoing the trauma of accepting they have the disease and the side effects of conventional cancer treatments. With skill and sensitivity this method supports expression, release and self-regulation in a gentle way (see Case study 6.1).

Case study 6.1

The following dialogue is feedback that the author received from a patient who had breast cancer, a year after completion of therapy. (Note: P = psychotherapist.)

P: *What role do you think I played in helping you with your early stages of cancer treatment?*

Anna: *I appreciate the care and support you gave during my cancer treatment and that I could talk to you about my problems. The weekly massage and breath work helped me to relax and get back into my body.*

P: *What did you find most helpful in our work together?*

Anna: *I could explore issues with you that I could not share with anyone else. Also I felt that you were right there with me, every step of the way, listening to me and supporting each step I took in my recovery. Even when I was feeling very depressed and ill during chemotherapy, your commitment and gentle encouragement helped me to keep going. You never gave up on me. That was important. In the later work when I learnt to release my childhood emotions, the messages in my body, I learnt to trust myself and access my emotions and feel safe and free to have my emotions. That was amazing when I learnt to do that.*

P: *What do you believe caused your cancer?*

Anna: *Possibly an early life with a terrified mother which put my body into a state of chronic stress. Also my low self-esteem and deep sense of helplessness and isolation. Probably unexpressed fear that I held for my mother.*

P: *What do you believe were the psychotherapeutic issues we dealt with that have kept your cancer at bay?*

Anna: *I believe that by dealing with my issues that I have become far more confident and healthy in every sense. I lead a very different lifestyle now, enjoy myself more and have some good, close friends. I have read that a tumour takes approximately 8 years to obtain its own blood supply and reach a stage where it can be detected. The article suggested that a patient might find it helpful to examine their lives 8 years prior to their diagnosis. In my case after my marriage ended, I experienced a period in which I questioned the reason to live more than at any other time. I believe that I was at such low ebb that my immune system was compromised. In my work with you I learnt to accept and love myself.*

The most important aspect of working as a body psychotherapist is the understanding and use of the therapeutic relationship. One aspect of the therapist's role is to hold the therapeutic relationship/space rather like a crucible, and to use curiosity and awareness to overview and support a patient's intra-psychic processes. Another aspect of the role is to 'enter into the cruci-ble', and be one of the elements in the mix. This enables working with inter-personal processes and how these reflect and affect the intra-psychic process within the patient. Open communication with the psychic and somatic trans-ference and counter-transference that occurs between the therapists and patient is practised. Transference has been described by Greenson (1991) as the 'experiencing of feelings, drives, attitudes, fantasies and defences toward a person in the present which are inappropriate to that person and are a repe-tition, a displacement of reactions originating in regard to significant persons of early childhood' (p. 33). Counter-transference has a number of meanings; Kottler (1993) identifies that it can be used to describe several responses, including 'as a reference to all the feelings a therapist has towards a client, as the therapist's reactions to a client's transference, or as the therapist's own transference feelings toward a client' (p. 116). Counter-transference can be experienced physically by the therapist, which Eiden (2002) has described as 'somatic resonance'. The therapist tunes into his or her own emotional responses and 'uses this resonance as counter-transference to address the client's inter-nal process' (p. 46). This concept in also discussed in Chapter 5.

Working with these processes to inform the open communication is enabled by the therapist tracking signals (for example, verbal and non-verbal – kinaes-thetic and visual – in particular fine movements). Once identified, this infor-mation can be used to process what is evolving between therapist and client. The observations can be used to form a basis for dialogue between therapist and patient. Alternatively, the therapist can wait for things to emerge in the patient, the therapist, or in the relationship. This mix can create the environ-ment that supports what is trying to emerge for therapeutic change. Questions such as 'What is it that releases the tension for my patient, and for the thera-pist?' 'What is the patient's unmet need?' and 'What moves us to our authentic selves and self-regulation?' need to be asked.

BODY PSYCHOTHERAPY METHODS

Table 6.1 lists some of the methods used in the author's practice of body psychotherapy. When a patient is first introduced to body psychotherapy methods, the rationale behind each technique is explained. The start point is usually relaxation and awareness activities to help individuals learn how to attune to their body and to familiarise them with this way of working. During this early phase open communication contracts are established. This includes a channel for safety so that the therapist knows that he will receive feedback about a patient's feelings of safety. When the patient has learned to work with the therapist in this way, then the work can move into a more experimental phase, which may involve touch, voice, and movement work. Family members and friends of people with cancer may also present for body psychotherapy (see Case study 6.2).

Table 6.1
Body psychotherapy methods

Method	Psychotherapist's task	Patient's task
Philosophical guidelines	The psychotherapist recognises that: People are born okay People in emotional difficulties are nevertheless full, intelligent human beings All emotional difficulties are curable, given adequate knowledge and the proper approach (Steiner 1974). The psychotherapist works with an empowering approach that enables patients to take responsibility for their life	To recognise that she is okay and are responsible for their therapeutic journey
Active listening	To provide a safe, attentive presence, and to promote open and honest contact To listen with acceptance, empathy and congruence (Rogers 1987)	To be open and to give honest feedback about the impact that the therapist (positive, neutral and negative) has on her
Contracting	To provide clear business and therapeutic contracts with patients (Berne 1966), which clarify ground rules and fit with Steiner's (1974) four requirements – mutual consent, valid consideration, competency and lawful object To check whether the patient's therapy contract is clear, is stated in positive words, and that it is possible, safe and observable and moves the patient through therapeutic change (Stewart 1989)	To agree to the guidelines, recognising that this will keep both the patient and the therapist okay and to be willing to keep open communication about the working progress
Working with psychodynamic processes	To notice, track and discuss these processes with patients: transference, counter-transference, projection, defensive, regression and resistance The therapist will analyse observations with his or her clinical supervisor and works with personal issues that may arise for his or her patients	To process the information that the therapist discloses

Self-awareness in the patient Focusing and tracking	To increase patients' awareness of internal processes the psychotherapist asks them to track what is happening in their body Open questions are asked such as: What do you sense, feel emotionally, see, hear, taste? What do you stop yourself from doing? How do you do that?	To stay interested in their own process, to experiment with awareness, to learn about sensations, reactions and impulses and to give feedback to the therapist To be able to feel more and to express these feelings in life when appropriate
Noticing	To help patients develop curiosity about how they function in relation to self and others, bodily observations are used for treatment direction. For example, the therapist notices where the body is immobilised, perhaps frozen in fear or anger. The patient learns how to relax that part of the body and move it again (see relaxation methods below). The psychotherapist notices where a group of muscles are chronically contracted or overly flaccid, and helps the patient release the contractions or mobilise the underdeveloped areas	
Self-awareness in the therapist	To bring somatic and counter-transference process into awareness, the psychotherapist uses focusing and noticing to track what is going on in his own body, and uses these sensations both as clues about what may be happening to the patient, but also to identify what is happening for the therapist. These may reflect counter-transference issues and it is possible that he may be picking up clues about what the patient is unable to express (authentic feelings). For example, the therapist may feel a sense of sadness while the patient is describing a sad situation while smiling	Patient works with the feedback from the therapist about somatic counter-transference
Grounding	The psychotherapist may use specific bioenergetic exercises (Lowen 1958) to help release and discharge energy and tension. The author prefers to use simple walking and Qi Gong movements, working alongside the patient (The metaphor of a tree with roots and a strong flexible trunk with a sense of expansion through the branches to describe the sensation and movement of energy through a grounded body can be useful in explaining grounding)	The patient practises these activities and develops a sense of different states of being, learning how to release and shift energy in the body

Table 6.1 continued over

Table 6.1
Body psychotherapy methods—cont'd

Method	Psychotherapist's task	Patient's task
Breath work	The psychotherapist introduces breath work activities to the patient. These can be used lying, sitting, standing, or in movement. As in grounding above, the therapist works alongside patients and demonstrates these activities to them Breath work is useful to oxygenate the body and to induce the relaxation response. Centring breath helps patients to stay mindful and in the present	The patient learns to attune to the body and develop a mindful approach. The patient uses breath to engage with, recharge, discharge and relax. This supports the natural rhythm and pulsation of the body
Relaxation therapy	Patients can be helped to learn about the concept of stress management and the physiology of the fight/flight/freeze/submit response. Kinaesthetic techniques are particularly useful. Patients are also asked to stay focused on these sensations in the present, and to let go of intrusive thoughts Patients may be asked to write a stress indicator diary	To practise relaxation techniques for 30 seconds up to 10 minutes several times a day to interrupt and manage habitual stress responses
Movement work Fine movement Release movement	Movement work helps to release 'blocked energy' and emotions The therapist tracks behavioural clues for the interrupted impulse, for example, if the patient moves forward and then stops. The patient is encouraged to process the movement or the resistance to it Patients may be asked to kick, hit outwards or move physically. They may be asked to increase their energy and deepen their breathing when this is appropriate to what is going on in therapy. Kicking the legs, for example, will increase the breathing rate and vitality to the legs, bringing out what a patient needs to kick about, e.g. kicking may lead to a release of suppressed emotion, such as rage or deep crying	With all these movement processes the patient experiments, moves and explores new senses of self, to increase expressive repertoire and develop a new intra-psychic perspective

Amplification and authentic movement (expressive movement)	The patient is encouraged to exaggerate movement or to move into a spontaneous dance. The therapist moves alongside the patient to support an emerging sense of self	The patient directs the process by working with open feedback and the effects of the contact
Touch for therapeutic reasons	The psychotherapist uses touch with the patient's permission, which can include: Placing one or both hands on the patient's back to ground and calm Massaging the patient's hands, feet or back to help relax or ground Experimenting with different types of touch to discover how the patient gives or receives Putting gentle pressure on either side of the patient's nose if she is holding back tears Holding a patient's hand while she is walking, to help her sense the ground, thus offering support to a shaky patient Holding the patient's head that has lacked very early support, or for the therapist to stand with his back against the patient's back, thus literally backing her up – or simply holding the patient. These actions are all done with the appropriate care	
Character analysis	Careful observation of how the patient's body is structured, how she carries herself and moves can be useful diagnostically, helping to understand the patient's core issue	Draw a body map to develop an understanding of the physical display of her core issues
Body mapping	For example: Are the shoulders hunched forward? Is the structure top heavy? Does the patient appear to have her feet on the ground or her head in the clouds? Is the body well developed or does it look like the body of a small child? Conclusions are drawn from observations about when trauma halted development and what kinds of defence are practised currently. For example, a heavily muscled body has probably been suppressed at a later time in life. Such a body has different defences and will require a different treatment strategy than a body that is underdeveloped and fragile	Collating this type of information is empowering for the patient Awareness is the key to change

93

Case study 6.2

Andrew, aged 38 years, was one of four brothers with a father who had been diagnosed as having liver cancer. Andrew had a difficult relationship with his father, who had rarely shown affection, and in his teens had been physically abused by him on a number of occasions. In his weekly sessions with the body psychotherapist, Andrew explored how the experience had affected his self-esteem and difficulties in receiving praise and gratitude from others (his work involved helping others and he had a tendency to overwork). Andrew wanted to connect with his father before he died. There was also anger and sadness for what he had gone through as a teenager.

During the 6 months of therapy, time was spent helping Andrew explore these feelings and his father's imminent death. Sometimes Andrew would express anger using cushions, which helped to release waves of sadness. The therapist used physical holding through a blanket to comfort Andrew at these times. This was negotiated with Andrew so that he was in control of receiving any touch. Andrew found gentle holding of his head and feet to be very helpful, as well as breath work to open his chest and vocal cords. Empty chair work was used to speak to his father asking for what he had wanted (and not wanted) as a teenager.

Andrew reported that the work had helped him feel okay about spending time with his father in the days before he died. He was able to sit quietly at his side, and even finally hold his father's hand, without reacting to an urge to walk away. His father had responded to this by saying, 'I am not proud about how I treated you when you were growing up, but I am proud of you and I wish I had more time to get to know my son'.

TRAINING, SUPERVISION AND INTEGRATING BODY PSYCHOTHERAPY IN CANCER CARE

According to William Cornell (1997) it is an essential ethical and clinical safeguard that any psychotherapist or counsellor using direct physical contact with patients is trained in, and responsive to, transference and counter-transference issues. Cornell argues touch can and often will evoke work for the patient to address, which if skilfully used, can correct such historical experiences and distortions as:

- Deprivation and neglect.
- Over-stimulation, intrusion and bodily violation, or sexualisation.
- Parental narcissistic use of the child.
- Deadening of vitality and use of the body as an instrument.

Cornell (1997) believes these chronic historical distortions of body experience will emerge within *both* the bodily and the interpersonal processes in therapy, and the responsible therapist actively attends to both. Body-focused methods, especially the use of touch, are likely to evoke powerful transferential and counter-transferential processes.

Assisting patients (or their carers) to work through issues in adjusting to living with cancer can be very complex. Making sense of behaviours and responses, and negotiating with patients as to what they hope to achieve through psychotherapy, is not for the novice. As with any professional helping service, therapists require not only training and supervision for this work, but also a working knowledge of cancer and its treatment. Integrating body psychotherapy with healthcare settings will necessitate healthcare practitioners developing an understanding of this work. In time, closer working relationships can help to bridge the practices of mind and body interventions for the benefit of patients.

SUMMARY

The chapter has been an introduction to body psychotherapy. As yet there is a paucity of literature on body psychotherapy and cancer care. There is a need for research work to formally evaluate this clearly profound way of working with patients and carers. The work of the body psychotherapist has been succinctly described in 1991 by the European Association of Body Psychotherapists (see Box 6.2). It is suggested that this statement be a cornerstone of sensitive and skilled practice of body psychotherapy in cancer care.

Box 6.2

Directly or indirectly, body psychotherapists work with the person as an essential embodiment of mental, emotional, social and spiritual life. They encourage both internal self-regulative processes and the accurate perception of external reality. Through their work, body psychotherapists make it possible for alienated aspects of the person to become conscious, acknowledged and integrated parts of the self.

As voted on and accepted at 3rd Congress of European Association of Body Psychotherapists, Lindau (September 1991). Online: www.eabp.org

ACKNOWLEDGEMENTS

I am grateful to my therapist Sean Doherty for his skill as a body psychotherapist and to all of my trainers, in particular Nick Totton for his in-depth analysis and writings about body psychotherapy. I would also like to express my appreciation to William Cornell for his articles, which incorporate body psychotherapy thinking into the world of transactional analysis.

Appendix 6.1
Development of body psychotherapy (Young 1997)

Time scale	Practitioners/teachers influenced by Reich and the body psycho-therapies they developed
Reich's Norwegian period	
1930–1939	Ola Raknes, Gerda Boyesen, David Boadella, Paul Ritter, Lillemore Johnsen – Norwegian School
	AS Neill, a patient of Ola Raknes and friend of Reich's, influenced parents and teachers with his progressive theories and methods directly based on Reich's theories of early sexual and physical repression
Reich's American period	
1939–1957	Alexander Lowen and John Pierrokas, patients of Reich, developed Bioenergetic analysis
	John Pierrokas included psycho-spiritual component to develop Core energetic therapy
	Charles Kelly – RADIX
	Myron Sharaf, patient and biographer of Reich's – Orgonomist
	Ellesswoth Baker – Orgonomist
Post-Reichian	
1970s	Fritz Perls, patient of Reich's who went on to develop Gestalt therapy
	Ida Rolfe – Rolfing
	Josef Heller, originally trained in Rolfing – Hellerwork
	Ron Kurtz – Hakomi
	Stanley Keleman – Somatic process

Appendix 6.2

Current body psychotherapies (mostly European and American)

Adapted from Totton (2003, pp. 88–115). In italics are the psychotherapist's questions, which help to differentiate between the different therapies.

Reichian therapies/post-Reichian and neo-Reichian

These therapies support that humans are naturally joyful, loving, creative and productive, that we are pulsating fields of energy, and become unhealthy when this pulsation is blocked. Free pulsation is impeded by repression of free expression and creativity in response to anticipated, perceived or actual social pressure and/or trauma. This pressure may occur in the past or present.

What is fixated and what needs to be freed in my patient?

Lowen and Pierrokas – Bioenergetics (Lowen 1976)
John Pierrokas – Core energetics (Pierrokas 1987)
Stanley Keleman – Somatic emotional therapy (Keleman 1987)
Charles Kelly – Radix (Kelly 1974)
David Bordella – Biosynthesis (Bordella 1987)
Gerda Boyesen – Biodynamic therapy (Boyesen et al 1980)
Lisbeth Marcher – Biodynamics (influenced by Johnsen 1976)
Ida Rolfe – Rolfing (Feitis 1978)
Josef Heller – Hellerwork (Heller & Henkin 1986)
Jack Painter – Postural integration (Painter 1984)
Peter Jones, William West, Nick Totton, Em Edmonson, Peter Armstrong –
    Energy stream (Totton & Edmonson 1988)
Nick Totton – Embodied relational therapy (Totton 2003)

Primal therapies

These therapies pay particular attention to the healing value of regression, the re-experiencing and abreacting of early deep traumas, in particular during infancy and childhood. The concept of body memory is particularly important.

What trauma is frozen in my patient and what needs to be re-experienced in order to be released and healed?

Arther Janov – Primal scream (Janov 1972)
Stanislav and Christina Grof – Holotrophic breathwork (Grof 1975; Taylor
    1994)
Leonard Orr – Rebirthing (Orr & Ray 1983)

Trauma therapies

These therapies draw on current neuroscientific thinking. They are used specifically with trauma work and post-traumatic stress disorder (PTSD).

What needs to be soothed to get the system back into balance?

Peter Levine – Somatic experiencing (Levine 1997)
Babette Rothschild – Somatic trauma therapy (Rothschild 2000)
Pat Ogden – Sensorimotor psychotherapy (Ogden & Minton 2000)

Process therapies

These therapies shift their focus from working with content to process. They recognise the importance of the past and of fixated states but the focus is on what is trying to change and grow without necessarily asking why this is happening or has happened. This group also draws on Chaos and Complex Theory, Buddhism and Taoism.

What is trying to emerge?

Fritz Perls – Gestalt (Perls et al 1973)
Arnold Mindel (Jungian analyst) – Process orientated psychotherapy (Mindel 1985)
Ron Kurtz – Hakomi (Kurtz 1990)
Eugene Gendlin – Focusing (Gendlin 1996)

Expressive therapies

These therapies focus on bodily expressive and creative aspects of the human being, specifically authentic and movement and voice work. They are also influenced by Carl Jung's concept of active imagination.

What is trying to be expressed?

Dance movement therapy with roots in Eutony, Gymnastik, Grindler work, Eurythmy (Johnson 1995). See also Chance (1975), Trudi Schoop (1974), Mary Whithouse (Chodorow 1991)
Albert Pesso and Diana Boyden-Pesso – Pesso Boyden system psychomotor (Pesso 1973)
Conrad Da'oud – Continuum movement (Conrad Da'oud 1995)
Alfred Wolfsohn – Voice and Voice Movement Therapy (Newham 1999)

REFERENCES

Berne E 1966 Principles of group treatment, 1994 edn. Shea Books, California
Bordella D 1987 Lifestreams: An introduction biosynthesis. Routledge and Kegal Paul, London
Boyesen G 1980 The collected papers of biodynamic psychology. Biodynamic Psychology Publications, London
Cameron R 2002 Subtle bodywork. In: Staunton T (ed) Body psychotherapy. Brunner-Routledge, Hove, East Sussex
Carroll R 2002 Biodynamic massage in psychotherapy: reintegrating, re-owning and re-associating through the body. In: Staunton T (ed) Body psychotherapy. Brunner-Routledge, Hove, East Sussex
Chance M 1975 Marion Chance: her papers. Edited by H Chaiklin. American Dance Therapy Association, Columbia
Chodorow J 1991 Dance therapy and depth psychology. Routledge, London
Conrad Da'oud E 1995 Life on land. In: Johnson DH (ed) Bone, breath and gesture: practices of embodiment. North Atlantic Books, Berkeley, CA
Cornell WF 1997 Touch and boundaries in transactional analysis: ethical and transferential considerations. Transactional Analysis Journal 27(1):30–37
Corr CA, Nabe CM, Corr DM 1999 Death and dying, life and living, 3rd edn. Wadsworth, Belmont, CA

Dreher H 1995 The immune power personality – 7 traits you can develop to stay healthy. Plume/Penguin, New York

Eiden B 2002 Application of post-Reichian body psychotherapy: a Chiron perspective. In: Staunton T (ed) Body psychotherapy. Brunner-Routledge, Hove, East Sussex

Feitis R 1978 Ida Rolf talks about rolfing and physical reality. Excerpts from Dr Rolf's early class lectures. Rolf Institute of Structural Integration, Boulder, CO

Gendlin ET 1996 Focusing-orientated psychotherapy. Guilford Press, New York

Greenson R 1991 Techniques and practices of psychoanalysis. Hogarth Press, London

Grof S 1975 Realms of the human unconscious. Souvenir Press, London

Heller J, Henkin WA 1986 The body work book: gaining maximum use and pleasure from your body. Putnam, London

Janov A 1972 The new primal scream: primal therapy twenty years on. Cardinal, London

Johnsen L 1976 Muscular tonus and integrative respiration. In: Boadella D (ed) The wake of Reich. Coventure, London

Johnson DH 1995 Bone, breath and gesture: practices of embodiment. North Atlantic Books, Berkeley, CA

Kastenbaum RJ 2004 Death, society, and human experience, 8th edn. Allyn Press, Boston

Keleman S 1987 Embodying experience: forming a personal life. Center Press, Berkeley, CA

Kelly CR 1974 Educating in feeling and purpose, 2nd edn. Radix Institute, Santa Monica

de Kooker M 2001 Psychoneuroimmunology – an overview. Online. Available at: www.wellness.org.za/html/pni.html

Kottler JA 1993 On being a therapist. Jossey-Bass, San Francisco, CA

Kübler-Ross E 1999 On death and dying. Routledge, London

Kurtz R 1990 Body-centered psychotherapy: the Hakomi method. LifeRhythum, Mendocino

Levine PA 1997 Waking the tiger: healing trauma. North Atlantic Books, Berkeley, CA

Lowen A 1958 The language of the body. Collier, New York

Lowen A 1976 Bioenergetics. Penguin, Harmondsworth

Mindel A 1985 Working with the dream body. Arkana, London

Newham P 1999 Therapy: the practical application of voice movement therapy. Jessica Kingsley, London

Ogden P, Minton K 2000 Sensorimotor psychotherapy: one method for processing traumatic memory. Traumatology (Online journal) 6(3). Available at: www.fsu.edu/~trauma/v6i3/v6i3a3.html

Orr L, Ray S 1983 Rebirthing in the new age. Celestial Arts, Berkeley

Painter JW 1984 Deep bodywork and personal development: harmonising our bodies, emotions and thoughts. Center for Release and Integration, Mill Valley

Perls F, Heffer RF, Goodman P 1973 Gestalt therapy: excitement and growth in the human personality. Penguin, Harmondsworth

Pert C 1997 Molecules of emotion. Simon and Shuster, Sydney

Pesso A 1973 Experience in action. New York University Press, New York

Pierrokas J 1987 Core energetics: developing the capacity to love and heal. LifeRhythm, Mendocino

Reich W 1973 The cancer biopathy. Farrar, Straus and Giroux, New York

Rogers CR 1987 Patient-centered therapy. Constable and Co Ltd, London

Rothschild B 2000 The body remembers: the psychophysiology of trauma and trauma treatment. Norton, New York

Schoop T 1974 Won't you join the dance? National Press Books, Palo Alto, CA

Steiner C 1974 Scripts people live: transactional analysis of life scripts. Grove Press, New York

Stewart I 1989 Transactional analysis counselling in action. Sage Publications, London

Totton N 2003 Body psychotherapy – an introduction. Open University Press, Maidenhead

Totton N, Edmonson E 1988 Reichian growth work. Prism Press, Dorset *This book is no longer in print. You can download it from http://www.erthworks. co.uk/*

Taylor K 1994 The breathwork experience: exploration and healing in non-ordinary states of consciousness. Hanford Mead, Santa Cruz

Young C 1997 Body psychotherapy: its history and present day scope. Online. Available at: http://www.eabp.org

FURTHER READING

Ader R, Felten DL, Cohen N (eds) 1991 Psychoneuroimmunology, 2nd edn. Academic Press, San Diego

Black PH 1995 Psychoneuroimmunology: brain and immunity. Scientific American: Science & Medicine Nov/Dec, pp. 16–25

USEFUL ADDRESS

Sue Hampton
Co-director of bodysense@work ltd
Website: www.bodysenseatwork.co.uk

Therapist as teacher

7

Peter A Mackereth, Jacqui Stringer and Diane Gray

Abstract

Massage as a therapy usually happens when the therapist provides the treatments to patients. There may be times, however, when it is more advantageous to the patient for massage to be provided by a carer or for a patient to learn self-massage. This chapter examines how, when and why professional therapists need to develop their skills with regard to teaching and supporting parents and carers to provide massage interventions. It also includes some issues relating to the legal aspects of working with infants and children. Case studies are utilised to illustrate how therapists can enable parents and partners to provide safe and therapeutic massage. Prophylactic abdominal massage (PAM) training for patients with leukaemia is also discussed to exemplify the potential health benefits of self-massage techniques.

KEYWORDS

involvement, empowerment, teaching skills, learning styles, safety, supervision, support

INTRODUCTION

The practice of providing massage in cancer care settings highlights the need for flexibility in who delivers the treatment. Therapists are not available 24 hours a day, so sometimes it can be more appropriate, and very valuable, for a family member or partner to provide touch techniques (see Chapter 8). Often, opportunities to teach others arise when parents and partners become interested in learning a skill that offers something positive to their loved one. It is not unusual for a patient's carers to feel hopeless and helpless. To be able to offer touch and massage, even in the form of a simple hand or foot massage, has benefits for both receiver and giver. The authors of this chapter have detailed strategies to help parents, partners and patients learn the gift of massage.

TEACHING ROLE AND EXPECTATIONS

In most situations, the therapist will be helping adults to learn new skills so that they can be used competently and confidently for supporting a loved one. Parents/carers might perceive the therapist as 'the expert' and believe that they will be unable to match the therapist's level of skill and apparent ease of delivery. Thus therapists will need to change their approach from being 'the expert' therapist to one of 'teacher/facilitator'. It will help all therapists who find themselves in this new role to have some understanding of the adult carer as a learner, the teaching/learning styles available, and the processes involved in helping someone acquire a new skill.

Furthermore, when recruiting therapists to work in healthcare settings, employers may include knowledge and experience of teaching skills as requirements of the post. Therapists may need to consider continuing education to develop skills in mentoring and teaching the art and science of their professional practice, if these were not already included in their undergraduate training (see Chapter 4).

LEARNING STYLES

Even though parents and carers may not know much about the theory and practice of massage and touch techniques, they will bring to any learning situation their own preconceived ideas and strongly held beliefs. Adults may not have been in a learning situation for years where they have been motivated to learn something new under stress or pressure. They may be hesitant and lack confidence as they do their best to get the skills and the sequences 'right'. Adults may perceive the therapist as 'the expert', and may compare their levels of skill to those of the therapist. Parents and carers need to learn quickly so that they can see the benefits straightaway; time may be short and the need to be helpful urgent and important. There will be an expectation that the therapist will be competent in helping them learn and will show respect and encouragement for their efforts. Feedback is more likely to be appreciated when it is given in a constructive and non-judgemental manner.

Honey and Mumford (1992) adapted Kolb's (1984) original Learning Styles Inventory, and identified four stages in the learning process:

1.   Activist – having an experience.
2.   Reflector – reviewing the experience.
3.   Theorist – concluding from the experience.
4.   Pragmatist – planning the next steps.

Honey and Mumford (1992) demonstrate how individuals favour particular stages and tend to pay less attention to aspects of learning. Most adults will be unaware of what has become their preferred learning style, and therapists may not be aware that both they and the parents/carers may have different ways of applying themselves in a learning situation. Typically, but not exclusively, activist carers may actually ask if they can 'have a go' and work along-side the therapist. Reflectors will want to watch closely and will be curious about the process and techniques involved. If the potential 'carer' student is a theorist he or she will prefer handouts, and structured teaching sessions – ideally on a one-to-one basis. The ever practical pragmatist may already have done some massage training, and will have been watching and learning very attentively. Pragmatists are eager, but they like structure and instructions that are unambiguous and have an obvious practical application. An outline of the learning styles is given in Box 7.1.

Box 7.1
Learning styles

Activists want to get on with the task, without considering what they really want to learn and what they need to know, and do, in order to learn the skills. When interested, they will join in the learning session enthusiastically, although they may have to be encouraged to reflect on how the quality of what they do can be improved. Activists learn best from active involvement and learn least from handouts, watching and direct lectures. These learners will want to work alongside the therapist. Therapists may need to 'rein them in' by using breaks to stop and reflect.

Reflectors usually ponder and question rather than jump in to learn new skills. Reflectors can get distracted by detail and may think of many different ways of doing the massage, rather than the endpoint, i.e. giving the massage. They will want to observe and re-observe, and have time to digest what they have seen. They like to hear about research and the massage experiences of other carers and the patient. In practice, this may mean they will be cautious and need space to work out how and when they want to learn.

Theorists gather information before they attempt a task. They like very structured and directed ways of working. They learn best from activities that follow a logical sequence, including lectures and demonstrations. Theorists learn least from unstructured spur-of-the-moment activities, without the aim being clearly articulated. They may be uncomfortable in a group situation, where feelings or unplanned-for contributions may arise. Well-presented handouts, which include theoretical information, will be welcome and reduce wariness of trying something new.

Pragmatists like to set clear goals, which is easy to do so long as they can recognise a practical application. They may be intolerant of the theoretical aspects of a situation and are usually focused and keen to achieve their goals. They like to pay attention to detail and have good organisational skills. They may need support in situations where there is no right answer. Pragmatists like to be involved in practical activities and learn least from theoretical lectures and unstructured activities with no clear purpose.

When in a teaching role, therapists need to be aware of what they can do to make it easier for learners to maintain their attention and involvement. For example, a parent or carer could be asked if they would like to sit closer to watch a technique; written information such as 'Simple Massage Techniques for Parents/ Carers' could be made available; or the parents/carers could be invited to participate in a structured teaching session later. They could also copy the massage strokes on their own arms/hands as a first step. The feedback may then be helpful in guiding the therapist in planning individualised teaching. If this interaction occurs in the presence of a patient, it will also be important to note and consider his or her responses to the questions posed. The therapist must be sensitive to the patient's wishes. Patients may be enthusiastic or reticent about whether or not the parent/carer is involved in the giving of the massage or the touch techniques.

INVOLVING CARERS IN PROVIDING MASSAGE

Given that cancer predominately affects adults, the therapist is likely to come across situations where 'carers' other than parents (i.e. partners, family members and close friends) may show interest in providing massage to a patient. It is not unusual to meet carers who have taken massage training and are already providing treatments at home; many therapists have begun their careers by practising with friends and family. However, this training may not have been of sufficient depth to enable them to skilfully treat a patient who is experiencing symptoms such as fatigue, extreme weight loss, breathlessness or clotting disorders. Offering to teach a carer massage may not be appropriate if the individual would feel overwhelmed by performing such a personal and intimate activity. For similar reasons, a patient may not want massage from a carer. An important rule for any therapist is to assess the situation and take cues from both the carer and the patient. The therapist may offer an easy 'opt out' by saying, 'I can come back another time' or 'So you can have some space to think about it'. Case study 7.1 describes a powerful experience of the effects of teaching simple massage to a carer.

Case study 7.1

Denis was visiting his life partner, John, who had throat cancer. John was recovering in a hospital ward after surgery. Denis confided in the ward's massage therapist that he was worried about showing affection to John by holding his hand in front of other visitors and patients. The therapist suggested she teach Denis foot massage as a practical way of relaxing and comforting John. Both John and Denis were keen for this to happen. Over the next few days, the therapist demonstrated techniques on John's hands and feet. At first, Denis watched and then joined in, mirroring the techniques on the opposite foot and then on the opposite hand. After watching for a while, a patient's son in the opposite bed asked the therapist if she would teach him to massage his father's feet. During her next visit to the ward, the therapist noticed Denis happily chatting to other visitors in the bay, holding his partner's hand.

Teaching massage to parents: evidence, concerns and safety

In many cultures, such as in India, massage of infants and young children is a normal part of life. In the West, awareness of baby massage and its benefits are increasing, but there is still a long way to go before it becomes a part of every new life (Glover et al 2002). There is a wealth of research into the benefits of teaching baby massage in a community setting (Bond 2002), which can be a useful resource for teaching these skills to parents in hospital settings. Some of these studies have focused on the father providing the massage. Cullen et al (2000) recruited fathers to provide their infants with daily massages 15 minutes prior to bedtime for 1 month. By the end of the study, the fathers in the massage group were more expressive and showed more enjoyment and warmth during floor-play interactions with their infants.

Dr Tiffany Field and her team at the Touch Research Institutes (see Chapter 3) conducted a number of disease-specific massage studies where parents provided the massage treatments. In a study by Field et al (1997a), children with asthma (n = 32; 16 4–8-year-olds and 16 9–14 year-olds) were randomised to a massage or relaxation group. The parents (male and female) were taught to provide one therapy or the other for 20 minutes prior to bedtime, nightly for 30 days. Compared with the relaxation group, the younger children showed an immediate decrease in behavioural anxiety and cortisol levels after massage, and the older children reported lower anxiety after the massage. In another study by Field et al (1997b), children with mild-to-moderate juvenile rheumatoid arthritis received massage from their parents 15 minutes a day for 30 days (a control group participated in relaxation therapy). In comparison with the relaxation group, anxiety and stress hormone (cortisol) levels were immediately decreased by massage. Over the 30-day period children's self-reports, parent reports, physician's pain assessment (both the incidence and severity) and pain-limiting activities all decreased. Specific to cancer care, Field et al in 2001 studied the effects of daily massage therapy given by parents to children with leukaemia (n = 20) compared with standard care (control group). After a month of massage therapy, depressed mood decreased in the children's parents, and the children's white blood cell and neutrophil counts decreased.

LEGAL AND PRACTICAL CONCERNS

Fearon (2005), a complementary therapist and children's nurse, has reviewed complementary and alternative medicine (CAM) use in paediatric services and suggests that concerns in the recent past have inhibited integration and necessary research work. These observations are supported by Wall (2002) (see Box 7.2), who have suggested that on the whole, NHS trusts have been suspicious of complementary therapies. The trusts are concerned about the legal and financial implications of vicarious liability and employment law when massage is practised and taught by NHS trust employees. Litigation is

> **Box 7.2**
> **Recommendations for safe practice (adapted from Wall 2002)**
>
> - The techniques taught should be ones that are nationally approved.
> - The interventions should be tried and tested and have outcomes that have been documented.
> - The parent/carer should be observed using the techniques.
> - The parent/carer should fully understand what is being done and why.
> - The parent/carer should know when to stop using the technique.
> - The parent/carer should know when to ask for help.
> - Clear written instructions along with diagrams should be given.

a growing healthcare cost and given that claims can arise many years later in cases involving infant and children, policies and practices are carefully scrutinised, with medical and nursing records being kept for several years after the provision of treatments.

In the need to ensure the best for children, both healthcare professionals and parents are understandably cautious about any additional interventions. Parents may also seek complementary and alternative treatment in the belief that these approaches can be both helpful and 'natural'. This perspective is not without its problems as many CAM interventions lack evidence of efficacy and safety, particularly in the area of herbal medicines (Ernst 2004, Fearon 2005). For example, there are times when massage will require careful adaptation or be unhelpful. Therapists and parents must be aware of these situations. Massage should not be given when the infant has a rash or broken skin, shows negative cues (e.g. does not settle to it or becomes distressed), or has been fed within the previous 1 hour. In children and adolescents with haematological disorders such as leukaemia, providing gentle massage would be subject to agreed practice guidelines approved by the clinical team (see Chapter 9).

The teacher also has a duty of care to ensure the safety of both parent and patient during the teaching session and in relation to any guidance given on massage. It needs to be recognised that health and safety checks, as well as risk assessments, are an important part of the legal requirement of all complementary therapists (Stone 2002). Any criterion that needs to be addressed should be investigated before any session takes place. The Health and Safety at Work Act (1974) states that the primary objective for the management of risk should be to remove or reduce the risk by proactive rather than reactive management. There is always potential to cause harm and therefore therapists must always be aware of health and safety issues. When practising, the therapist should audit their practice and any resources used (e.g. recommended/supplied oils and creams, towels, handouts and recommended books), thus providing a base for further improvement of the service for their learners (Wall 2002). Therapists need to be acutely aware of who has to consent to the therapist's touch and massage when working with any child or young person.

There is also the important safety issue for the therapist, who is a stranger to the child and family. In healthcare and other services for children, such as teaching and nursery care, all staff are screened before having access to children and vulnerable adults. A police check of criminal records is one part of that process, supervision of staff is also essential. The authors recommend that massage of young children is performed only when parents are present (ideally by the parent(s) themselves), with clear and observable permission of the child. Children must be supported in making a choice and must fully understand that they can ask for the touch to stop at any point. Therapists could demonstrate the strokes using a child-sized doll, or another consenting adult, in full view, so that the child can clearly see what is being offered. The clinical team responsible for childcare must be in agreement with regard to provision of complementary therapies, and be consulted prior to treatment or massage training being offered.

Agreeing a standard for teaching massage to laypersons is important, as parents may be concerned about their abilities and potential to do harm. Infant massage instruction standards again can be a useful starting point. Wall (2002) points out that registered massage instructors do not have the right to give the impression or assurance that only they know what is best for the patient or a parent. In addition, parents are consenting to being shown how to provide massage to their baby with the therapist demonstrating on a doll and providing close supervision. Therapists should be registered with a regulatory body, so that they are accountable, adhere to a code of conduct, and hold indemnity insurance. The public must be able to complain and have access to relevant information pertaining to the therapist's fitness for practice and professionalism. Two such bodies exist in the UK: the Guild of Infant and Child Massage and the International Association of Infant Massage. In addition to the recommendations for safe practice it is also essential that therapists protect the integrity of their work by:

- Keeping detailed records of their work with children and parents (according to the hospital/community trust policy and Data Protection Act 1998).
- Reporting any concerns about the physical and psychological wellbeing of the child.
- Working with children only in the presence of their parents.
- Ensuring they have the written permission.
- Obtaining consent from consultants and/or nursing staff, especially if the child is receiving medication.

WORKING WITH INFANTS IN CANCER CARE

In the first year of life cancers are extremely rare and largely confined to neuroblastomas, retinoblastomas and hepatoblastomas. These are examples of embryonal tumours, which result from faulty development of cells resembling fetal tissue (Thompson 2001). Advising and providing infant massage instruction in this context would be complex, and if considered, must be carefully supervised by therapists with both health professional status and training in teaching infant massage. Tipping (2005) suggests that gentle containment holds may help to provide parents with physical contact and comfort, without destabilising a fragile and sick infant.

Teaching massage to a mother, who is herself living with cancer, may also be possible. Women in their fertile years are sometimes diagnosed as having cancers such as leukaemia or breast cancer, yet little has been reported about interventions that might be helpful to the mother and child relationship (Kirsch et al 2003). Not only are they mothers, but also patients having to consider aggressive forms of cancer treatments. Breastfeeding would not be appropriate and symptoms such as fatigue, immuno-compression and low platelet counts may make it difficult for them to have quality time or to play with their child. Case study 7.2 describes a remarkable scenario when Kelly, a young mother who delayed her treatment to give birth, was isolated in a leukaemia unit. Kelly was able to learn infant massage, which provided quality time with her baby while she was receiving cancer treatment, which was intense, and at times, debilitating.

Case study 7.2

Kelly was diagnosed as having acute myeloid leukaemia during the second trimester of her pregnancy. Rather than risk the life of her child, she decided to continue with the pregnancy and undergo treatment after the delivery. The fatigue and reduced immunity from the illness and medical treatments limited Kelly's time with her baby. Infant massage instruction was offered as an opportunity for her to bond and have quality time with her baby and enjoy giving nurturing touch. The experience of baby massage also helped Kelly to relax. The therapists provided the instructions over three short sessions using a doll and then visited Kelly to support her while she provided 10 minutes of massage to her baby each day with brief breaks. As Kelly's health improved, for a while she was able to increase the massage time to 15 minutes without a break. Kelly and her family were very grateful for this teaching and support, and commented on how relaxed she and the baby were after each session.

WORKING WITH CHILDREN AND ADOLESCENTS

As described earlier Dr Tiffany Field and colleagues have reported numerous quantifiable benefits of teaching parents to massage their children. Therapists and parents have also made anecdotal comments to the authors of this chapter about how this intervention can have wider implications for the health and wellbeing of both parent and child (see Box 7.3). There is a need to build on the work of Dr Field and others by formally auditing, evaluating and researching the practice and outcomes of the teaching of massage to parents and carers in cancer care settings. Anecdotes and research evidence aside, therapists need to be mindful of the immediate concerns of parents of a child living with cancer before offering either massage or training in massage skills.

When a child or adolescent is first diagnosed with cancer, this can be devastating for all concerned, as parents do not expect to hear that their child has cancer (Thompson 2001). Fear can be a major factor in limiting physical contact for some parents. Teaching and supporting a parent to carry out technical care activities is now advocated by healthcare professionals, and important in valuing their contribution and expertise in a child's care

---

Box 7.3
Potential benefits of teaching massage to parent(s)

Benefits for the parents

- Massage helps support permission to touch, and is a potential source of pleasure, relaxation and enjoyment.
- Massage builds and maintains a strong parent–child bond during illness.
- Learning massage helps parents to relax with their child at a traumatic time in their lives.
- Both parents can feel involved, emotionally and physically, in their child's care.
- Giving massage promotes quality time and offers quality activity for parents.
- Massage is a physical activity that also has health benefits for the massage giver.

Benefits for the child

- Maintenance of good muscle tone and co-ordination is encouraged.
- Recuperative sleep can be promoted at a time when the illness, treatment and hospital admissions can increase fatigue and disrupt normal sleep.
- Massage can assist in boosting and supporting the immune system.
- A closer bond between parent(s) and child can be developed.

(Lipman 2001). For example, a parent might learn to administer medication via a nebuliser or change simple dressings. However, a parent's anxiety can inhibit learning, with concentration on instructions and guidance compromised by worry and tiredness. Teaching massage at the bedside can also be complicated by interruptions for necessary medical and nursing reasons. It also needs to be acknowledged that some young patients may prefer to receive massage from a health professional rather than from a relative or partner.

Adolescence can be a time when teenagers try to seek independence from their parents (Thompson 2001), so having 'comforting' contact with a parent might not be acceptable, particularly in front of others. Another option, recommended by Field (2000), is to involve a grandparent. Not all young people reject contact with their parents, so it is important to take the lead from the patient. It is also important to avoid stereotyping when offering to teach parents from diverse cultural and social backgrounds (Sheikh & Gatrad 2001) as practices and customs may vary across generations and within cultural/social groups (see Case study 7.3).

Case study 7.3

Zaheer, aged 15 years, had advanced cancer and his condition had deteriorated with cerebral metastases. He insisted on the curtains being closed as the light hurt his eyes and increased his headaches. His mother spent much of the evening sitting quietly in his room. She divided her time between the hospital visits with spending what time she could with her other children (aged 7 and 9 years). Zaheer showed no interest in massage until his mother agreed to receive a session herself in his room. The therapist then offered to treat Zaheer. He agreed, and she gently worked on the reflexology areas for the head, eyes and neck as part of a 20-minute massage to his feet and hands. Zaheer's mother watched every movement closely. Massage was something that his mother had done for Zaheer when he and his siblings were infants.

Zaheer reported to his nurse that his headache had eased and he had slept better after the treatment. On visiting him the next day, the therapist found Zaheer's mother massaging his feet while being guided by her son. The therapist offered to help Zaheer's mother learn some reflexology techniques. With her consent, the therapist worked with mother and son for three sessions until she was sure that Zaheer's mother was confident of providing a 15-minute treatment. By the end of the week Zaheer was telling his mother that she was as good as the therapist in easing his headache and helping him sleep – she beamed on hearing him say that.

TEACHING PATIENTS TO USE PROPHYLACTIC ABDOMINAL MASSAGE

Patients suffering from the haematological malignancy acute lymphoblastic leukaemia (ALL) receive, as part of their initial or induction therapy, a drug called vincristine. Vincristine is one of a family of drugs known as the vinca alkaloids, which are used to treat ALL, lymphomas and some solid tumours such as breast cancer. Like all forms of chemotherapy they cause side effects, and neurological toxicity is a common feature of treatment with all vinca alkaloids. However, this is the dose-limiting side effect of vincristine; in other words, patients may have the drug dose reduced or the drug omitted from their treatment regimen if the side effects are too bad. The neurological toxicity usually manifests itself as either peripheral neuropathy causing 'pins and needles' or numbness of the extremities (more commonly the feet are affected) or autonomic neuropathy. (Note: similar symptoms occur in patients with myeloma on treatment protocols that include either thalidomide or bortezomib (Velcade®).)

Autonomic neuropathy can present as abdominal pains, extreme bloating and constipation. Although the nervous system will usually recover fully, the recovery is slow. If the effects are severe, as suggested above, dosage of vincristine will be reduced and in some cases omitted. Consequently, this side effect can lead to suboptimal treatment. It can also cause the patient a great amount of discomfort, sometimes for up to 2 weeks or more. Current prophylaxis against the related effects of 'vinca bowel' relies on laxatives. This course of action is sufficient in some cases, but patients with severe problems are subject to an intensive course of 'bowel clearing' through oral preparations, suppositories and enemas. Unfortunately, such solutions cause added discomfort and distress to the patient. They are not always successful and in the case of enemas or suppositories there are the added dangers of bleeding (due to low platelet counts) and trauma/perforation of the bowel.

An initiative aimed at tackling this problem has been commenced on the Adult Leukaemia Unit (ALU) of the Christie Hospital NHS Trust, Manchester, UK. The scheme consists of administering gentle prophylactic abdominal massage (PAM) to all ALL patients from when they are first admitted for treatment until the last dose of vincristine has been given (a maximum of 6 weeks). PAM is given two to three times daily, usually in the hour before meals. PAM is typically carried out using base oil incorporating a blend of essential oils. It has been introduced into the routine care of these patients as a supplement to normal laxative prophylaxis, not as an alternative. The patient, and where possible, an appropriate family member, are explained the rationale for offering PAM training. They are then taught the PAM routine (described below) by example. The patient/carer is then observed performing PAM and monitored on a regular basis by the therapist, who also documents the efficacy of the massage in maintaining gut motility. The information given to patients and the massage routine is given in Box 7.4 (a–c). See also Case study 7.4.

Box 7.4
PAM information leaflet

(a) Why massage your abdomen? (Figure 7.1)

- Constipation can be a side effect of one of the chemotherapy drugs in your treatment (vincristine).
- Constipation can also occur due to dehydration, poor diet, having limited mobility or through taking certain analgesic drugs.
- This gentle massage is a supportive and preventative measure rather than a substitute for medical treatments, such as laxatives.

(b) Ten PAM steps

1. Wash and dry hands.
2. Apply oil supplied by therapist.
3. Place cupped hands over tummy (Figure 7.2a).
4. Circle tummy in a clockwise direction using both hands (×6) (Figure 7.2b).
5. Scoop down left side of tummy using the heel of your hand (×6) (Figure 7.2c).
6. Scoop up starting on the lower right side, then move across your tummy finishing down the left side, following the large bowel (×6) (Figure 7.2d).
7. Circle tummy clockwise again (×6).
8. Stroke with fingers of alternate hands up the right side of the tummy, from the start of the large bowel, across the tummy then down the left side (×6) (Figure 7.2e, f).
9. Repeat the clockwise circles (×6).
10. Finish by gently holding the tummy with cupped hands.

(c) Points to remember

- Always use clockwise movements.
- Only use gentle pressure; if any discomfort, stop and seek advice.
- Use the massage before a meal, rather than immediately afterwards.
- It is recommended that you perform this massage twice a day.
- Ideally the massage should be carried out with the patient lying down. If this is not possible, it can be done with the patient semi-prone.
- Try to avoid interruptions.
- Take your time and be relaxed.

Tips to avoid and manage constipation

- Ensure good fluid intake as much as possible. Check the recommended amount with your nurse or doctor.
- Continue to take prescribed medication.
- Maintain mobility if possible.
- Seek nutritional advice from dietician.
- Use the abdominal massage to help prevent and manage constipation.

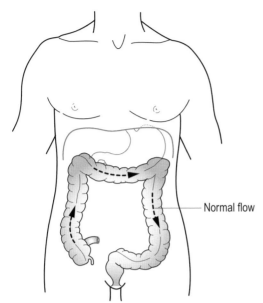

Normal flow

Figure 7.1   A diagrammatic representation of the large bowel showing the direction of normal flow of contents.

Case study 7.4

Christine was a young woman who gave birth in October 2003 and was diagnosed with acute leukaemia in January 2004. The nurse therapist met Christine soon after she was admitted. She was found to be suffering from biphenotypic leukaemia, which apart from having a poor prognosis also meant she would be given vincristine as part of her treatment. The possible side effects of the drug were explained. The nurse therapist demonstrated PAM on her own body, and as Christine followed the instructions, the benefits were discussed. The next time Christine was visited she cheerfully said that she had been performing the massage three times a day, with each session lasting 15 minutes. Her bowel habit was regular. It was gently explained that she did not have to massage for so long (typically PAM takes about 5 minutes). She smiled broadly and stated it was her comfort blanket. The astonishing thing about Christine was that she went through her whole treatment without taking any laxatives (they are usually given prophylactically) while maintaining a very regular bowel habit throughout. She gained so much comfort from the massage that she continued it long after the vincristine was stopped.

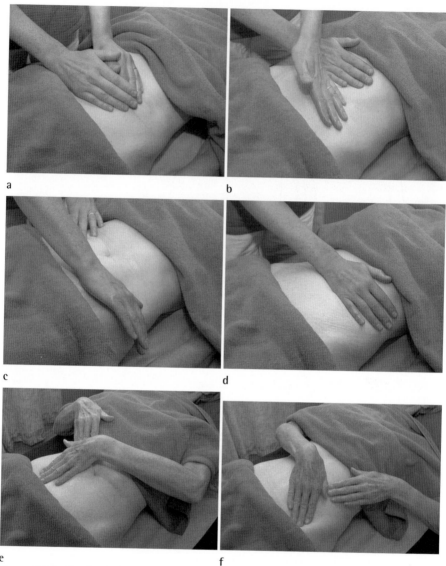

e   f

Figure 7.2 (a–f) Prophylactic abdominal massage. See Box 7.5 for details of the steps of the massage.

Although these techniques are currently being offered to ALL patients, other patient groups (including the myeloma patients mentioned earlier) are at risk of developing similar problems. These and other patients are likely to benefit from such interventions. For example, any patient who requires opioids will be susceptible to chronic constipation. PAM offered to patients at the time of initial prescription of problem drugs could prevent or minimise such side effects.

> ## Box 7.5
> ## Recommendations
>
> - There is a need for therapists to develop their skills and confidence in facilitating and sharing massage skills with others.
> - Parents/carers of children should have the opportunity to learn and practise simple and safe massage routines and techniques.
> - Carers of adult patients may be offered teaching sessions and/or opportunities to carry out touch therapies alongside a qualified therapist.
> - Care must be taken not to impose massage training on carers, given the burden and stresses of caring.
> - An important element of learning massage skills is experiencing receiving and sharing what feels comfortable and helpful.
> - Patients can be taught self-massage and reflexology techniques to help with symptoms and build-on sessions provided by qualified therapists.
> - Teaching activities need to be evaluated and audited to gather information about its limitation and benefits and improve teaching packages.
> - There is a need to produce good quality videotapes and instruction leaflets to supplement, but not replace, skilled teaching and ongoing support.
> - There is a need to audit, evaluate and research formally the practice and outcomes of teaching parents/carers/patient massage in cancer care settings.

SUMMARY

This chapter has examined the role of the teacher/facilitator in recognising and working with individuals who have different learning styles, with regard to beneficial touch techniques. There are many benefits of involving parents and carers in giving massage. However, it is important to acknowledge that parents/carers may not want to carry out massage and/or may be too over-whelmed by the experience of caring for someone with cancer to consider it. It also needs to be recognised that patients' responses to involving their family can range from embarrassment to enthusiasm. Examples of projects teaching massage to parents and patients have been given to illustrate the potential benefits and issues when considering offering massage training in the clinical setting. Recommendations for developing best practice in this important work are listed in Box 7.5.

ACKNOWLEDGEMENTS

Liz Tipping and Tina Green.

REFERENCES

Bond C 2002 Positive touch and massage in the neonatal unit: a British approach. Seminars in Neonatalogy 7:477–486

Cullen C, Field T, Escalona A et al 2000 Father-infant interactions are enhanced by massage therapy. Early Child Development and Care 164:41–47

Ernst E 2004 Herbal medicines for children. Clinical Pediatrics 42(3):193–196

Fearon J 2005 A reflective overview of complementary therapies for children 1995–2005. Complementary Therapies in Clinical Practice 11(1):32–36

Field T 2000 Touch therapy. Churchill Livingstone, London

Field T 2003 Touch. The MIT Press, Cambridge, MA

Field T, Henteleff T, Hernandez-Reif M et al 1997a Children with asthma have improved pulmonary functions after massage therapy. Journal of Pediatrics 132:854–858

Field T, Hernandez-Reif M, Seligman S et al 1997b Juvenile rheumatoid arthritis: benefits from massage therapy. Journal of Pediatric Psychology 22: 607–617

Field T, Cullen C, Diego M et al 2001 Leukaemia immune changes following massage therapy. Journal of Bodywork and Movement Therapies 5(4): 271–274

Glover V, Onozawa K, Hodgkinson A 2002 Benefits of infant massage for mothers with postnatal depression. Seminars in Neonatology 7(6):495–500

Health and Safety at Work Act 1974

Honey P, Mumford A 1992 The manual of learning styles. Peter Honey, Maidenhead

Kirsch D, Sallie E, Brandt PA et al 2003 Making the most of the moment: when a child's mother has breast cancer. Cancer Nursing 26(1):47–54

Kolb DA 1984 Experiential learning. Prentice-Hall, Englewood Cliffs, NJ

Lipman TH 2001 Hospitalized children with chronic illness: parental caregiving needs and valuing parental expertise. American Journal of Maternal Child Nursing 26(6):344

Sheikh A, Gatrad AR 2001 Muslim birth practices. The Practising Midwife 4:410–413

Stone J 2002 An ethical framework for complementary and alternative therapies. Routledge, London

Thompson J 2001 The needs of children and adolescents. In: Corner J, Bailey C (eds) Cancer nursing: care in context. Blackwell Science, Oxford

Tipping L 2005 Adapting touch techniques: the neonate. Connections 1(9):6–8

Wall A 2002 Agreeing a standard for infant massage: not a soft touch. Journal of Neonatal Nursing 8(3):93–96

FURTHER READING

Daines J, Daines C, Graham B 1998 Adult learning, adult teaching. Continuing Education Press, England

Fleming Drehobl K, Gengler Fuhr M 2000 Pediatric massage: for the child with special needs. Therapy Skill Builders, USA

McClure V 2003 A handbook for loving parents. Bantam Books, New York

MacGregor J 2000 Introduction to the anatomy and physiology of children. Routledge, London

USEFUL ADDRESSES

The Guild of Infant and Child Massage
22 Elder Close
Uttoxeter
Staffordshire ST14 8UR
UK
Tel: 07796 916179
Website: www.gicm.org.uk

International Association of Infant Massage
Christine Allen
40 Silk Mill Road
Redbourne
Hertforshire AL3 7GE
England
Tel: 01582 791933
Website: www.iaim.org.uk

Teenage Cancer Trust
Website: www.teenagecancertrust.org

Practitioners at work

Section contents

INTRODUCTION

Section 1 explored key themes related to the underpinning evidence, theoretical basis and clinical practice of massage and bodywork approaches in cancer care settings. Section 2 focuses on the professional practice issues related to specific clinical areas of innovative developments. The contributing authors have sometimes written as teams, which reflect the collaborative nature of the work. The practice areas discussed, although not exhaustive, are exemplars of evolving and valued work by therapists.

In each of the nine chapters in this section the authors overview the intervention(s) and consider the key issues and concerns in developing the practice within their clinical area. Reflective accounts, anonymous case studies and the available literature are used to examine practical concerns and issues. Recommendations are made for best practice and further development.

To start with, in Chapter 8, The HEARTS process, Ann Carter describes how different techniques drawn from massage, bodywork and aromatherapy can be combined to form a simple, yet profound approach. The effectiveness and application of the techniques are demonstrated through case histories. Chapter 9, Massage and essential oils in haemato-oncology by Jacqui Stringer, describes the challenges involved when introducing a complementary therapy service in a protective isolation unit following high-dose cytotoxic chemotherapy, total body irradiation, or blood and marrow transplantation for the treatment of haematological cancers such as leukaemia or lymphoma. Case histories are used to illustrate the roles that massage and essential oils have played in patient care. In Chapter 10, Collaborative working, Karen Livingstone and Anita Mehrez illustrate the benefits of a combined therapeutic approach in the management of symptoms of breast cancer treatment. The origins and development of this approach is described to illustrate how professionals can work together to provide a model service.

Chapter 11, Shiatsu for symptom management by Jill Bailey, describes the origins of shiatsu and the principles on which it is based. Indications and contraindications are discussed and reference is made to traditional use of floor work and the merits of adapting treatments through the use of a massage chair. The purpose of Chapter 12, Managing lymphoedema by Cheryl White, is to increase understanding of the nature of the condition, and to establish an awareness of the complexity of lymphoedema treatments. Optimising patient care through collaborative working is discussed and key issues for the massage therapist, including contraindications and ways of adapting massage treatments, are described. In Chapter 13, Massage and spinal cord compression, June Rosen and Joanne Carr describe the project developed in response to a request for patients for foot massage. As patients with this condition often present with reduced distal sensation a major concern for the therapist is not doing any harm. The service was initiated from a partnership between two physiotherapists, with one working as a complementary therapist.

Chapter 14, Creative approaches to reflexology by Edwina Hodkinson, Barbara Cook and Peter Mackereth, reviews the theories and practice of reflexology, clarifies concerns and then describes innovative approaches to safely adapt treatments for patients and the carers in cancer care settings. In Chapter 15, Adapting chair massage, Gwynneth Campbell, Peter Mackereth and Paola Sylt explain how chair massage is becoming increasingly popular in the workplace and other social settings. They explore and describe a project set up to provide the intervention in cancer care to patients, carers and staff. More specifically the authors report on findings from service audit and evaluation of a carers' service. Lastly, in Chapter 16, Being met with care: massage work with vulnerable patients, Nataly Lebouleux and Ann Carter explore the development and maintenance of the therapeutic relationship. The context in which the therapist works is described with the emphasis on working with vulnerable patients living with cancer. Recommendations are made identifying ways in which therapists can work sensitively with vulnerable individuals.

8

The HEARTS process: combining therapeutic approaches for relaxation

Ann Carter

Abstract

HEARTS is an acronym for 'Hands on', Empathy, Aromatherapy, Relaxation, Textures and Sound. The aim is to help patients and carers to easily achieve a state of relaxation and feeling of wellbeing. HEARTS always involves physical touch and empathy, and relies largely on the involvement of the patient and the intuition of the therapist, rather than set techniques. This chapter describes the origins of the process and the rationale on which it is based. Case studies are used to demonstrate how the different elements may be used to create a flexible therapeutic approach. Situations where HEARTS has been particularly useful are explained, with attention drawn to adaptations for particularly vulnerable patients. Recommendations are made at the end of the chapter.

KEYWORDS

intuition, relaxation, imagery, empathy, sound, textures, touch

INTRODUCTION

HEARTS ('Hands on', Empathy, Aromatherapy, Relaxation, Textures and Sound) is a combination of techniques which can be used at all stages of the cancer journey, for patients as well as for carers and staff. The approach was devised at the Neil Cliffe Cancer Care Centre in Manchester where the author was working as an aromatherapist and facilitator for a relaxation and massage group for patients. The individual aromatherapy sessions usually lasted for an hour; most patients found them enjoyable and much benefit was gained. However, the author felt that in some circumstances the use of essential oils, bases and creams was not the best use of therapy time or the therapist's expertise; such situations are outlined in Box 8.1.

Box 8.1
Situations where aromatherapy was felt not to be the most
appropriate approach

- Where patients had advanced cancer, poor co-ordination, friable skin or poor muscle tone, conventional massage techniques were often less appropriate.
- Patients who were very ill could only receive aromatherapy massage for a short time. Something needed to happen 'in the moment' and in setting up the aromatherapy treatment, the 'moment' quickly passed.
- Some patients who wanted aromatherapy had symptoms such as jaundice, hyperventilation and profuse sweating, which are traditionally contraindicated for aromatherapy massage.
- Patients wanted to relax and sometimes, because they found this difficult, it was more comfortable to talk, rather than to avoid 'failing'.
- The therapist/patient wanted something more than foot and hand massage, especially where this treatment had been received on several occasions.
- Concerns were expressed that residual oil could come through clothes.

WHAT ELSE COULD BE HELPFUL?

The first source of inspiration for a combined approach came from two lines of the poem 'Break, Break, Break' by Tennyson:

> But O! For the touch of a vanish'd hand
> And the sound of a voice that is still.
>
> *Cited in Touch – an Exploration (Norman Autton 1989, p. 108)*

Through using her experience of different approaches to massage, body-work and relaxation techniques in many different settings, the author had noticed three key factors that can help promote relaxation:

- Whichever massage or bodywork technique is used there is potential for a state of relaxation to be achieved.
- Most patients are able to respond to the sound of the human voice during relaxation/creative imagery sessions.
- Even in a noisy and crowded environment, when touch and empathy are involved, a patient can still achieve a state of relaxation.

To overcome some of the difficulties in Box 8.1 a new therapeutic approach was considered. Criteria are listed in Box 8.2.

The question 'What gives enjoyment and pleasure, which will facilitate a state of relaxation?' was then posed. Some of the ways that enjoyment and pleasure can be achieved are through the approaches shown in Box 8.3.

Box 8.2
Criteria for new therapeutic approach

- The natural systems of the body would be encouraged to respond, e.g. the parasympathetic nervous system and the ability of the brain to release endorphins.
- The patient would remain clothed or covered to promote feelings of security. This would also avoid patients with poor co-ordination and/or those who have cachexia having to undress.
- The approach would be used easily on a busy ward as well as in a separate treatment room.
- The treatment could be simple and quickly effective as some patients can be still only for a short length of time.
- A combination of therapeutic approaches could be utilised to bring about rapid relaxation.
- The aim would be to 'treat' the person, i.e. to find an approach which the patient would find pleasurable and relaxing.
- The processes used would easily be taught to carers, therapists and healthcare professionals as a development of skills which they were already using in caring, nursing and therapy.

Box 8.3
Potentially enjoyable ways of giving and receiving touch and diverting the mind

Physical contact

- The hands-on work is given from a state of 'pali' which means 'loving kindness' (from Thai massage).
- Effleurage (stroking movements) from Swedish massage for relaxation.
- Holding techniques from healing modalities and craniosacral therapies.
- Finger brushing (the use of the fingertips, often used as a 'finishing stroke'.
- Palming and the gentle use of pressure from Thai massage and shiatsu.
- Textures of clothes and covers to help create a pleasant sensory experience (Thai massage and shiatsu are offered through clothes).

Mind-diverting techniques

- Touch is used to help the patient access kinaesthetic experience by encouraging the mind to refocus on the body, thus diverting the mind's constant 'inner dialogue'.
- Imagery techniques which can involve the patient's sensory experiences.

The following section provides an in-depth description of the six components of HEARTS and the role each one plays. Three elements, hands-on work, empathy and involving the textures of clothes and covers, are normally included in each treatment. Aromatherapy and the sound of the human voice can be offered, in addition, to help patients achieve relaxation.

'HANDS ON': WORKING WITH THE SKIN AS A SENSORY CANVAS

Massage is an ancient healing art which usually involves stroking and kneading techniques to relax underlying muscles. An oil or cream lubricant (which may have moisturising properties) is applied directly to the skin so that the therapist's hands can glide easily and the therapist can work easily at different depths. In HEARTS, the skin is regarded as a sensory canvas on which the hands, working as 'brushes', can 'paint their art'. The sensory canvas of skin is an organ with weight, a large surface area and extraordinary sensory capacities. These properties are outlined concisely in Box 8.4.

The skin is more innervated in certain areas of the body, the hands, face and feet being particularly well supplied with sensory receptors. With such a sensory network available to send messages to the brain, the author suggests that it is likely that skilful touch can be applied to small areas of the body to achieve a calming response. The sensory receptors are remarkable at detecting the minimum of sensation and change. The smallest of changes in temperature, textures and pressure can all be distinguished. For example, while walking, a

---

Box 8.4
The structure of the skin

The surface area of the skin has an enormous number of sensory receptors receiving stimuli of heat, cold, touch, pressure and pain. A piece of skin about the size of a quarter contains more than 3 million cells, 110–340 sweat glands, 50 nerve endings and 3 feet of blood vessels. It is estimated that there are some 50 receptors per 100 square millimetres, a total of 640 000 sensory receptors. . . . The number of sensory fibres entering the spinal cord by the posterior roots is well over half a million. The surface area of the skin is approximately 19 square feet in the adult male in whom it weighs 8 pounds, containing some 5 million sensory cells, the skin constitutes some 12 percent of body weight.'

Montague (1986, p. 7)

A quarter refers to a quarter dollar, about the size of a British 10 pence piece.

grain of sand can be detected in a shoe and a biscuit crumb can be detected by a patient in the bed; individuals who have their eyes closed can detect the differences between the textures of velvet, silk and cotton. The skin is sensitive enough to detect a gentle breeze or a minute change in temperature – although no physical contact has taken place.

Factors which may affect the ability to receive 'kind' touch

The degree to which patients feel able to receive touch may depend on their touch history. When sensory receptors are stimulated, nerve impulses are transmitted to the brain where they may be related to earlier experience. Some patients may have been stroked and cuddled as babies and children. They may have had their hair played with, their foreheads stroked, or their bodies massaged. Bath times may have been loving, fun occasions. Family and friends may have played touch games such as 'This little piggy went to market', or messages may have been 'written' on the child's back with a finger. Touch is an essential part of human development. Leboyer (1977) described touching and caressing a baby as food for the infant. He also recognised that when babies are deprived of this 'food' that they may fail to thrive and may even die as a result.

Therapists need to be aware of the emotional power of the hands to convey nonverbal messages of empathy and safety, as well as caring and, where appropriate, affection. For some patients, who are not used to receiving kind, respectful touch, the initial contact alone may create an emotional response. Some areas which may be particularly vulnerable include the abdomen, throat or upper chest. Some patient responses to receiving HEARTS are given in Box 8.5.

However, not all touch is good touch. For some patients, touch may have been manipulative and conditional, or associated with violence and abuse. These situations may make patients wary about what the therapist is offering.

Box 8.5
Patient responses

'That was absolutely gorgeous. I have never, in my whole life, experienced anything like it.'
'I never thought I could feel so good although I am so ill.'
'It's the best sleep I have had for ages.'
'I feel that I have more room in my body, The cancer doesn't seem so important any more.'

Where patients have been deprived of positive caring touch, some individuals may experience 'skin hunger' and really value what HEARTS can offer to them. An example is given in Case study 8.1.

Case study 8.1

Agnes, aged 84, received some over-all body stroking while wrapped in warm towels after a bath. With a big smile on her face she said, 'I've waited 80 years for this!'.

What had happened to the patient between the years of 4 and 84 is unknown. However, it is interesting that something so simple as stroking though towels should bring about such a profound response.

To facilitate touching patients in a caring way, HEARTS uses the concept of a touch library as a resource. A touch library may be defined as infinite ways of touching someone which brings about either a pleasant or relaxing experience.

There are many ways of touching someone. Five of the main strokes from the HEARTS library are:

- Stroking – along the body or in circles with the aim of relaxation.
- Finger brushing – for light work and a pleasant sensory sensation.
- Holding techniques – for stillness.
- Gentle pressure – for safety.
- Therapeutic holding – for tuning into tissues.

More than one therapist can work on a patient/carer at a time and this work can be pleasant to give and receive (see Chapter 14).

The strokes described above are not an absolute in themselves. Each stroke can be varied by the speed the therapist uses, the pressure applied, the length of the stroke, the area of the body covered, the rhythm, and the texture of the fabric through which it is applied (see p. 131). The strokes used can be agreed before the session starts so that the patient remains in control of the hands-on work (see Chapter 16). One of the first patients to experience the stroke library from HEARTS was Sam. His story is outlined in Case study 8.2.

> ## Case study 8.2
>
> *Sam, aged 54, had advanced cancer. He was in good spirits although his mobility was slow and his co-ordination poor. During the initial consultation, Sam requested aromatherapy massage for his back, head and shoulders with a 1% blend of lavender (Lavendula angustifolia) in sweet almond oil. He took 15 minutes to undress, and although he said he was comfortable when prone, turning to a supine position on the couch was difficult. His skin was friable and his muscle tone was slack. The oil blend seemed to sit on the surface of the skin. The treatment time was curtailed as the therapist realised it would take some time for him to redress. For the second and subsequent sessions, Sam was supported with pillows in a seated position with his legs under the massage couch. He was wrapped in a large warm towel and two drops of lavender oil were put onto the towel so that his body heat would aid its evaporation. The therapist used slow stroking movements though the towels, light pressures, palming from Thai massage and very gentle brushing movements. After receiving this treatment for about 15 minutes in complete silence, Sam said, 'That were grand!'. The therapist continued to work on his arms, neck, shoulders and head through the towels. Sam said he was better able to sleep at nights and both he and his wife felt more rested.*

EMPATHY

Empathy is a process which is fundamental to all therapeutic relationships. Mitchell and Cormack (1998) suggest that the empathy which is established between the therapist (practitioner) and a patient is able to transform the state of patients, so that their own inner healing resources can be mobilised. Rogers (1957) describes empathy as 'accurate understanding' and considers it to be part of a triad which supports conditions for change. (The other two components of the triad are 'unconditional positive regard' and 'openness'.) In practising HEARTS, empathy facilitates the use of intuition and creativity on the part of therapist and patient, so that each component can be applied in harmony with another, thus producing a synergistic effect.

In HEARTS, **touch and empathy** are fundamental and intertwined, one cannot be offered without the other.

Silent messages are given and received through the sensory receptors of the therapist's hands or as June Rosen, physiotherapist at Christie Hospital, said in private conversation, 'Hands are very eloquent if they are allowed to be'.

In Box 8.6, McFarland (1988) considers his approach to working with a new patient.

> ## Box 8.6
>
> 'Which of the countless massage, reflexive or deep tissue techniques do I apply to Cynthia? The truth is, I do none of these. I don't adjust Cynthia, what I do is Cynthia, Simply Cynthia. Every system at its very best is only an approximation of how to Cynthia. No single system can encompass a Cynthia. Each does have a piece, a very lovely piece to be sure, but it is not the package and we need it all to complete Cynthia...
> The work itself must derive from Cynthia.
> So the very best system of all... is to listen... and then Cynthia
>
> *McFarland (1988, p. 87)*

AROMATHERAPY

Aromatherapy may be defined as 'the systematic use of essential oils to improve physical and emotional wellbeing' (National Occupational Standards 2002). The use of essential oils from plants can play a useful part in stimulating the smell memory; pleasant memories can be evoked by using one or two drops of a patient's favourite essential oil on a tissue or on a towel. As the oil evaporates the aroma can enhance the patient's experience of receiving touch. Qualified and experienced aromatherapists who are on the organisation's Register of Practitioners (House of Lords Report 2000) can prescribe and mix suitable blends for use in HEARTS, although they may not be involved directly in the hands-on work. In this respect HEARTS offers opportunities for integrated working (see Chapter 2).

RELAXATION

Many patients learn to live with a state of stress and tension, unaware that the body has its own rebalancing capabilities which can be achieved through relaxation. Ryman (1995) has described relaxation as 'a state of consciousness characterised by feelings of peace, and release from tension, anxiety and fear' (p. 3). When a patient enters a relaxed state it is more than 'doing nothing'. The frequency of the brain waves are lowered from 14 cps (cycles per second) to 8 cps. The patient enters a day dream state which is similar to the state experienced when first waking or just before sleep. The relaxed state is the opposite of the 'high alert' or fight/flight which occurs when the stress response is activated. Some patients may have tried numerous relaxation techniques with varying degrees of success, and some may have given up completely. Suggestions for helping an individual to relax while using touch are given later in the section on sound. One patient told the author that he was unable to relax as he could not 'control the thoughts in his head'. However, when the therapist used a combination of touch and a simple refocusing technique, he was able to relax completely and enjoy the experience. See Case study 8.3.

Case study 8.3

Brian, aged 43, was an engineer. Although he had advanced metastatic spread, he was still working and he felt that he really needed to relax. He didn't want the therapist to use oil as he was going on to a business meeting. He lay fully clothed on the couch with his eyes wide open, his arms and hands clenched by his side. His legs were straight out in front of him, and his toes pointed to the ceiling. The therapist asked him what would be most useful to do in the next half an hour. He replied, 'I just want to relax, but I don't know how. My mind is so full of everything'. The therapist reassured him that his body still knew how to relax, it was just that his mind was getting in the way. She suggested that she could hold his head and in doing so she could pay some attention to the thoughts, so they would feel taken care of. Then she asked Brian to take his attention away from his head to his feet. She talked him through a very simpli-fied relaxation where she asked him to think of the space between different areas of his body. Within 2 minutes Brian had closed his eyes and his breathing became slower and deeper. The therapist decided to use a mix of holding and gentle pressures for the rest of the session (about 20 minutes). On completion, Brian looked a different person. His complexion was pink instead of white, his posture was more open and he looked rested. His body had remembered how to respond when the calming activity of the parasympathetic nervous system was enabled.

TEXTURES

Textures play an important role in HEARTS. Sanderson et al (1991) discusses the role sensory stimulation can play in the rehabilitation of adults with learning difficulties. Using this principle, the author decided that rather than regarding dressing gowns, sheets and covers as unessential, their textures could be used to enhance the hands-on sensory experience. A patient could be covered with a warm towel or soft blanket. These offer different textures through which the patient can experience touch, and at the same time create feelings of security. Every time a therapist changes the texture through which she works, the patient is able to receive a different sensory experience. Variations can be made in consultation with the patient. An example of where textures used to enhance the experience is given in Case study 8.4.

Case study 8.4

Martin, aged 45, was a keen sportsman who had been diagnosed with cancer 2 weeks previously. He was having intensive chemotherapy and spent some time on a near-by ward. When he felt too weak to walk to the treatment room, the therapist worked with the patient on the ward. He was able to adopt a semi-supine position supported by pillows. Martin's favourite oil was lavender (Lavendula angustifolia) and, when requested by the patient, the therapist used one drop of the oil on a tissue. The therapist worked sitting on the side of Martin's bed. She covered him with warm towels and worked with finger brushing and gentle pressures on Martin's hands, arms and head for 10 minutes. Martin liked the warmth and the mix of roughness and softness of the towel's texture. Still keeping contact with the patient, the therapist talked Martin through some imagery that he had designed. This involved visiting a garden with a variety of aromatic plants, many colours, and the sound of children laughing together with feelings of contentment. At the end of the session, Martin said, 'That was tremendous, I feel so much better'.

It is important to recognise that this session took place on a busy ward that was very noisy. A 'sacred' space can be created anywhere, providing that there is the will of the therapist and patient to create their own space amid the noise.

SOUND

This section refers mainly to the sound of the human voice. Therapists often rely on external sources of music to promote relaxation, and forget that their own voice can be a valuable and creative resource. Incorporating the use of the human voice together with 'vanished hand' (see quotation on p. 124) the patient can be helped to achieve relaxation. For some patients, skilful touch, together with some easy diversions for the mind, can help a person enter a relaxed state more easily than a single therapy used on its own. It is as though the therapist is holding the space that links body and mind, so that the parasympathetic nervous system can be brought into action. As in all therapeutic interventions, the approach is agreed with the patient before the treatment starts. To help achieve this relaxed 'daydream' state, the therapist's voice assists the patients to refocus their awareness. A script is not necessarily required. When the therapist is truly tuned into the patient, the patient's own body can be used to indicate the sequence to follow. The key for the therapist is to speak in a natural conversational style, and in a slower manner, and lower tone. Details of three approaches are given in Box 8.7.

Box 8.7
Three suggestions for helping a patient access relaxation through the combined use of the therapist's touch and voice

(1) The therapist places her hands gently on an agreed part of the patient's body – usually the feet, hands, knees, shoulders or head. She asks the patient to identify how the contact of her hands feels. (Patients usually identify feelings of warmth, safety, pressure or calm.) A positive sensation, e.g. warmth, is agreed with the patient. This sensation can then be used in a simple mind diversion to help the patient achieve a feeling of relaxation. The therapist invites the patient to think of 'warmth' travelling, in sequence, to different areas of the patient's body whilst physical contact is maintained.

(2) The therapist places his hands on an agreed area of the patient's body as described above. He then invites the patient 'to become aware of my hands resting on your feet'. He then moves his hands to the next body area, e.g. the knees, and says, '. . . and become aware of my hands resting on your knees . . .'. He then continues in sequence, pausing to give the patient time to become aware of the contact of his hands and the area of the body on which they are resting.

(3) The patient is invited to think of a colour which represents something which is important to her, e.g. a sense of relaxation, calm or peace. (The therapist does not need to know what the colour is.) The mode of entry for the colour is agreed before the session starts and the therapist repeats one of the processes described in (1) or (2) above. The therapist suggests to the patient that the colour the patient chose could travel to areas of the body, bringing with it the property attributed to it. If the patient believes that a certain colour (perhaps blue) represents peace, then as the colour travels round the body it brings peace to the areas it reaches, until the whole body is feeling relaxed and calm.

These mind diversions are very simple and they can help the patient (or carer) to refocus their thoughts on pleasant sensory experiences. Carers can easily learn these techniques, which can be used at home, or when a therapist is not able to give the treatment. (See Chapter 7, Therapist as teacher, p. 107.)

APPLICATIONS

HEARTS has been used on several occasions where patients have been particularly distressed, or where they have been very tentative about receiving a touch therapy. It has been used where patients have been very anxious, where they are unable to sleep, or where they are about to be moved from a ward to a hospice, or where a panic state is present. The latter is illustrated in Case study 8.5.

Case study 8.5

Emily, aged 65, had advanced metastatic malignant spread and was nearing the end of her life. The therapist was asked by a nurse if she would 'do some aroma-therapy' for Emily who was in a side ward. Emily was jaundiced, sweating pro-fusely and seemed to be hyperventilating, although she was wearing an oxygen mask. The therapist made the decision not to use essential oils and to find another way to alleviate her distress. The therapist sat on one side of the bed and told Emily that together they would do something to help her feel better. She put one of her hands on the top of the patient's crown and one hand on her abdomen. The therapist then suggested to Emily that she could feel relaxation coming from her hands and travelling through her body. Keeping one hand on Emily's crown, the therapist named the body areas she wanted to Emily to focus on in sequence. As she named each one, she put her hand on the area to make it easy for Emily to follow the progression. Shortly after starting the treatment, Emily's colour started to return. Gradually her breathing slowed, the sweating decreased, and after about 3 minutes Emily took off her oxygen mask and said clearly, 'Thank you, I feel much better now'. For the last few days of her life she remained calm and without the need for oxygen.

Therapists and healthcare professionals have also given some feedback about the results from using HEARTS. Some of their views are stated in Box 8.8.

RECOMMENDATIONS

The author believes that this simple, yet profound, approach could play a major role in many situations, especially as many healthcare professionals are already comforting patients by using touch, creating empathy and using a quiet voice when there is a need for reassurance. Recommendations for future develop-ments are given in Box 8.9.

SUMMARY

HEARTS relies on working with a mix of approaches to help calm and rebalance body and mind. It is a versatile and simple approach with wide-ranging bene-fits. A major advantage is that it can be used anywhere 'in the moment' and patients do not have to remove clothing. Patients who seem to find relaxation difficult seem to respond well to the combination of skilful touch and the human voice, and the experience is relaxing for the giver. HEARTS builds on existing skills used by therapists and healthcare professionals so it can easily be integrated into patient care.

Box 8.8
Feedback from therapists and healthcare professionals

'The results were much more profound than I dreamed of.'
'HEARTS is so easy to use, I use it most of the time now.'
'HEARTS has been so helpful. I wish I had learned it years ago.'
'When I don't know what else to say or do, I always have HEARTS. It has been invaluable.'
'It is so useful to have something to do at nights when patients wake up distressed. It helps to get them back to a relaxed sleep.'

Box 8.9
Recommendations

- HEARTS can easily be taught to carers and some patients.
- All therapists and healthcare staff should have the opportunity to learn this approach.
- HEARTS should be available to all patients, not just those with advanced illness.
- Referrals for HEARTS should be integrated into patient care in the same way as any of the other complementary therapies.
- There needs to be an in-depth evaluation of the benefits.

REFERENCES

Autton A 1989 Touch – an exploration. Darton, Longman & Todd, London

House of Lords 2000 Science and technology, sixth report, complementary and alternative medicine. HMSO, London

Leboyer F 1977 Loving hands. Collins, London

McFarland D 1988 Body secrets. Healing Arts Press, Los Angeles, CA, p. 87

Mitchell A, Cormack M 1998 The therapeutic relationship in complementary health care. Churchill Livingstone, Edinburgh

Montagu A 1986 Touching – the human significant of the skin. Harper and Row, London

National Occupational Standards for Aromatherapy 2002 Healthwork, UK

Rogers CR 1957 The necessary and sufficient conditions of therapeutic personality change. Journal of Consulting Psychology 21:95–103

Ryman L 1995 Relaxation and visualisation. In: Rankin-Box D (ed) The nurses' handbook of complementary therapies. Churchill Livingstone, Edinburgh

Sanderson H, Harrison J, Price S 1991 Aromatherapy and massage for people with learning difficulties. Hands On Publishing, England

USEFUL READING

Montagu A 1986 Touching – the human significant of the skin. Harper and Row, London

McFarland D 2000 Body secrets. Healing Arts Press, Los Angeles, CA, p. 87

Payne RA 2000 Relaxation techniques. Churchill Livingstone, Edinburgh

USEFUL ADDRESS

Ann Carter
Complementary Therapy Co-ordinator
St Ann's Hospice
Neil Cliffe Cancer Care Centre
Wythenshawe Hospital
Southmoor Road
Wythenshawe
Manchester M23 9LT
UK
Tel: 0161 291 2912
Email:acarter@sah.org.uk

Massage and essential oils in haemato-oncology

9

Jacqui Stringer

Abstract

This chapter describes the challenges involved when introducing a complementary therapy service on a protective isolation unit. Here, treatments can include high-dose cytotoxic chemotherapy, total body irradiation and stem cells transplantation for the treatment of haematological cancers such as leukaemia or lymphoma. The pathology of leukaemia is outlined along with symptoms that would normally contraindicate massage. Two case histories are used to illustrate the role that massage and essential oils have played in patient care and to illustrate some of the difficulties faced by patients with leukaemia. The origins of a project, which uses massage and essential oils as an integrated component of patient care, are described. A brief overview of the initial audit of the project is outlined, describing some of the successes of the service and user views. Recommendations are made at the end of the chapter.

KEYWORDS

haematology, leukaemia, lymphoma, choice, control, quality of life, massage, essential oils

INTRODUCTION

In high-dependency multi-modality treatment units, such as those treating patients with haematological malignancies, it is easy to focus on the administration of the various treatments needed to induce remission and support the patient with a range of medications. These include antibiotics, anti-viral and anti-fungal therapies, and blood product transfusions until the patient's immune system recovers. The primacy of care is to prevent and promptly treat the side effects of aggressive curative treatments and/or associated complications. There is a risk of nurses becoming so focused on ensuring that all interventions are delivered as prescribed – a science in itself – that they struggle to meet the patient's other needs. The expert haemato-oncology nurse becomes skilled at managing the frequent observations, administration of complex drug, blood and intravenous requirements so as to ensure the patient can maintain some quality of life during this prolonged period of hospitalisation.

With diseases such as leukaemia and lymphoma the patients can be almost ready for discharge at one minute but then develop a life-threatening infection and be dying from septic shock the next. Many newly diagnosed haemato-oncology patients only experience vague symptoms such as fatigue, lethargy and tiredness, perhaps bleeding gums or an infection which prompts them to go and see their general practitioner (GP). The GP takes a simple blood test known as a full blood count (FBC), the results of which bring the news of a life-threatening illness requiring immediate admission to hospital. The treatment required demands long periods of repeated high-dose chemotherapy to achieve remission and then finally stem-cell or marrow transplantation. At the time, a patient may be oblivious of what was causing these vague symptoms, and this obviously makes the diagnosis of cancer harder to bear. The speed of treatment is also difficult to comprehend; if left untreated, acute leukaemia can rapidly lead to life-threatening infections, bleeding and death. The lower the blood count at diagnosis the better the outcome. The treatment and outcomes of children and adults affected by leukaemia has improved over the past 20 years so it is no longer the automatic death sentence it was. The leukaemias are a group of blood cancers affecting the white blood cells, 'characterized by the malignant white cells in the bone marrow and blood. These abnormal cells cause symptoms because of: (a) bone marrow failure (i.e. anaemia, neutropenia, thrombocytopenia); and (b) infiltration of organs (e.g. liver, spleen, lymph nodes, meninges, brain, skin or testes)' (Hoffbrand et al 2001, p. 162).

It is possible to give an overview of the care, treatment and support patients receive in a high-dose therapy isolation unit (Figure 9.1). However, all patients are individuals and the same diagnosis seen in two patients can present differently from one to another. The type and sub-type of leukaemia come with specific treatments and prognostic outcomes, and equally, the age and gender of the patient, and the white blood count at diagnosis all influence the prognosis.

Being in the midst of so much technology and having to endure frequently changing physiological states can be frightening for the patient and their carers. For patients to feel safe, the healthcare professionals treating them must be people they can trust implicitly. Patients often feel they have no control over their situation and can feel very vulnerable. It is not always possible or appropriate for nurses to give patients a hug, something to 'make it better', even for a short time. However, this is often what is needed. Possibly, the most legitimate way of offering a therapeutic approach that involves deliberate kind touch is in the form of a massage. This must be from someone whom patients trust – an appropriately trained therapist who understands their condition and treatment.

HAEMATOLOGICAL MALIGNANCIES

Haematological malignancies, as previously discussed, are often difficult to identify as their associated symptoms can be very vague (e.g. fatigue). There are, however, a number of exceptions. These include lymphadenopathy (enlarged lymph nodes) in lymphoma patients and pathological fractures (bones breaking with minimal trauma) in myeloma patients – both of which cause obvious concerns regarding the use of massage. However, patients with haematological malignancies who are undergoing active treatment have many symptoms that are contraindications for massage; the commoner symptoms/side effects are shown in Box 9.1.

Box 9.1
Symptoms which are contraindications for massage

- Low platelet counts, with a potential for excessive bleeding and bruising.
- Vulnerability to infection due to minimal numbers of functioning white cells.
- Septic episodes.
- Hypotension.
- Tachycardia and rigors.
- Deep vein thrombosis.
- Erythematous rashes (which are frequently drug induced).

Due to the number of contraindications, massage services using essential oils have been developed at only a few haemato-oncology centres.

Despite the difficulties, and with the support of a medical team, such a service was developed in Manchester. Christie Hospital is a specialist cancer treatment hospital, which sees more than 12 000 new patients each year, mainly from the north-west of England. The aromatherapy massage service has been offered to patients of the 18-bedded adult leukaemia unit (ALU) since 1997. Each patient is cared for in an isolation room (Figure 9.1) while they undergo intensive chemotherapy often culminating in a bone marrow transplant.

INTEGRATING MASSAGE AND ESSENTIAL OILS INTO PATIENT CARE

When the new service started in 1997, the primary aim was to improve the quality of life of the patients on the ALU and that of their carers. This continues to be the main aim of the project, although 8 years later the author has become more ambitious about what may be possible. Realistically, it is impossible to alleviate completely the stress and anxiety of being on a leukaemia unit. However, some of the symptoms associated with stress, e.g. loneliness, insomnia, anorexia, depression and anger may be open to reduction (Cassileth & Vickers 2004, Field 2000, Hayes & Cox 2000, Hernandez-Reif et al 2004,

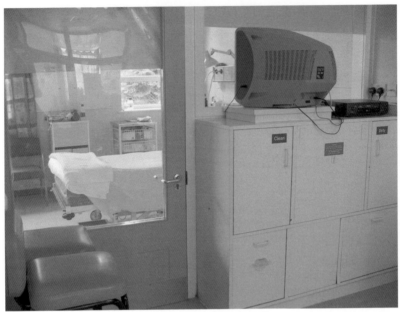

Figure 9.1 Isolation room on the adult leukaemia unit.

Post-White et al 2003). The aspiration of the service was to maintain patients' psychological 'status quo' and thus significantly reduce the need for psychiatric referrals, sleeping tablets, anti-depressants and anxiolytics. Massage is currently available two days a week, but it is hoped that in time it will become a daily service with all patients and carers having the opportunity to use it when they wish. One example of recent innovations within the service is the chair massage for carers, something which has proved to be very popular (see Chapter 15).

A secondary aim was to offer patients effective alternatives to the constant stream of drugs used to help alleviate side effects of the disease and the drug therapy. It may be that some patients feel most comfortable using conventional treatment for problems such as mucositis, constipation and nausea. In severe cases this approach is, of course, the most appropriate. Many patients, however, express a desire to reduce the amount of drugs they use. In the case of prophylactic medicine the reduction of drug use may be possible by using massage and essential oils in novel but appropriate ways. For example, abdominal massage has been used to prevent constipation, and antibacterial, essential oil mouthwashes may be shown to be an effective prophylaxis against infection due to mucositis. Feedback from patients suggests the latter have a better taste than most of the chemical-based ones used as standard. A practical angle to this argument relates to the financial implications, a couple of drops of appropriate essential oils in half a tumbler of boiled water used as a mouthwash would be far cheaper – as well as more pleasant – than large quantities of commercially produced mouthwash. From a clinical perspective, because of the small amounts required, it is possible that essential oils would also be easier on an overtaxed body than some of the conventional medications. When patients are admitted to the ALU they are stripped (metaphorically) of most facets of their normal life – clothes, home, work, loved ones, food and control over their environment. By necessity there is little that can be done about this. However, by offering choice wherever possible, patients can regain a limited amount of control over their lives; a fact that may be very important to their psychological wellbeing (Siegel 1986).

Case studies 9.1 and 9.2 will provide the reader with some understanding of the struggles patients may experience to survive and to give some insight into the gentle power of massage and the use of essential oils in such situations.

Case study 9.1

Kathryn, aged 35, was diagnosed with acute lymphoblastic leukaemia. She failed to go into remission straight away, and her leukaemia was brought under control. Kathryn received a matched unrelated donor (MUD) transplant 5 months later. This was the beginning of a very distressing stream of complications including life-threatening viral infections (through which she lost her sight almost completely), graft-versus-host disease (GVHD), including ulceration of the oral cavity. Kathryn passed away a year later having contracted yet another viral infection.

Understandably, through much of the last year she fluctuated between being withdrawn and openly distressed as she watched her body fade away and her legs and feet blow up with oedematous fluid. By nature, Kathryn was reserved and did not feel comfortable discussing her concerns with the medical team. She had shown interest in aromatherapy massage soon after her initial diagnosis and whatever problems she encountered she found relief through massage. Conversation was rare during her sessions, and she was often asleep by the end of the 20-minute treatment. Two sessions particularly indicate how significant massage was to her. The first was 2 months before her death when she was in acute renal failure. Although the doctors had consented to her receiving a massage, her father did not want us to proceed and tried to intervene. Kathryn got cross – and she received her massage! The second was on the day she passed away. Due to her viral infection her breathing was laboured, her oxygen saturations very low and she was visibly distressed. This time I had to persuade both the doctors and the nurses to let me see her. The look of relief on her face when I entered the room was heart warming. I used lavender and rose for her blend (her favourite oils) and spent most of the session using gentle holding techniques on her feet hoping to ground her and reduce her anxiety. By the end of the massage her breathing was calm and even, her saturations had gone up and she was asleep. She died a few hours later. To ease someone's passing in such a way is both an honour and the greatest blessing I could hope to receive for my work.

Case study 9.2

Mary, aged 54, was diagnosed as having acute myeloid leukaemia and requested to be transferred to Manchester for her transplant so as to be near her family. After having spent time in intensive care with pneumonia, Mary returned to the leukaemia unit. She was claustrophobic, suffering from nightmares and had not slept properly for over 2 weeks. She also had hypertension which the doctors thought may be due to chronic anxiety. They explained that Mary also had multiple thrombi; some in her left arm and some in her left calf. With such complications massage would not, under normal circumstances, be an option. With the support of the doctors, and after much thought, the therapist decided that she would work only on her feet and use holding techniques on the affected left side. At the time her blood biochemistry was completely deranged, so the therapist used only base oil for the session. Essential oils would have added too much of a burden to her obviously struggling liver and kidneys. The therapist spent her usual 20 minutes with Mary and at the end of that time she was fast asleep. Mary continued to sleep deeply for over 2 hours despite 'bleeping', monitoring, intravenous equipment and nurses coming in regularly to check her observations. Massage became a regular part of Mary's life. It helped her to sleep, keep her claustrophobia under control, her blood pressure stayed within the normal range and her feelings of anxiety were greatly reduced.

DOCUMENTATION

Before setting up the service, it was important to have the appropriate documentation in place. A list of essential documentation, devised for the service, is given in Box 9.2. Policies and guidelines were written for therapists who were using massage, with or without essential oils, for patients with haematological malignancies (leukaemia, lymphoma and myeloma). Because of the vulnerability of this patient group, it was imperative that clear guidance was available for all therapists regarding the relevant clinical issues.

Box 9.2
Service documentation

- Policies and guidelines for practice
- A doctor/patient written consent form
- Patient treatment record
- An audit form

Therapists require a thorough understanding of the illness, the medical treatments, as well as the physiological and psychological impact these have on patients. It is the author's personal belief that any therapist working in such a highly specialised unit should have statutory health professional status (e.g. as a nurse). Alternatively, the therapist must have gained related knowledge and have 2 years' prior experience of working in the field of oncology.

A doctor's written consent form, confirming that it is appropriate for a patient to be treated with massage, was devised for a member of the medical team to sign for each new referral. Once the form has been signed, it is shown to the patient as reassurance that the doctor(s) endorses the therapy. The patient and/or carer are then also asked to sign the form to confirm that they understand what is being offered.

The treatment record was developed from standard treatment sheets and was necessary in order to record a patient's history and to make notes regarding treatment sessions. There are now publications which offer sample copies of referral/treatment records (see Tavares 2003).

AN EVALUATION OF THE ALU PROJECT 1997/98

The service was audited from the outset. Patients were asked whether they were interested in taking up the offer of the service. Once they had received a massage they were encouraged to comment on the treatment they received. Finally, time was taken to network with healthcare professionals and therapists who had set up similar services in other hospitals. Unfortunately, there were very few people to contact at that time. Setting up the documentation proved to be a useful exercise in thinking through the processes involved. It helped to ensure that everything necessary was included and nothing of fundamental importance had been overlooked.

The ALU project started in spring 1997. Between April 1997 and December 1998, 92 patients requested massage and were treated. This is the equivalent to 26% of all patients admitted during this time (data source: the hospital's Business Information Officer). The audit form entailed the patient commenting (anonymously if they so wished) about the service and how appropriate it was to their needs. The audit also offered an opportunity for further comments to be made and recorded. The questionnaires were collected over the 18-month period; the patients' responses are discussed below.

Thirty-seven questionnaires were returned up to October 1998; all those responding said that they found the treatment beneficial. Some comments made by the patients included 'relaxing', 'therapeutic', 'eased pain', 'reduces stress', 'escape', 'tailored to needs' and 'slept well afterwards'. The only two 'negative' comments made were 'more frequent sessions please' and 'a longer session would be nice'. It appeared that the massage service had made a positive contribution to the services offered on the ALU. For example, 26 patients commented that the therapy was relaxing and soothing. In a time of high stress and anxiety, the massage service had made an important contribution to treatment and improved the patients' sense of wellbeing. Two patients noted specifically that massage eased their physical pain – without the aid of drugs.

FUTURE DEVELOPMENTS

In light of the positive audit results, it was felt that it would be appropriate to look at the specific benefits patients gain from the therapy. To this end, negotiations were undertaken with other professionals, which allowed the author to develop a research project assessing the effect of aromatherapy and massage on physiological parameters of stress. These were primarily measured through serum cortisol and prolactin levels, as well as looking for any impact on patients' perception of pain and their quality of life. The study was approved by the local ethics committee and had the backing of the Christie Hospital NHS Trust research and development department. Data collection for this study has now been completed and the results have formed the basis for the author's PhD thesis.

Alongside the clinical research, our laboratory work (contact author) has identified several essential oils, which, in vitro, are highly effective antimicrobial agents killing several clinically relevant and potentially fatal bacterial and fungal pathogens. This corroborates the findings of others, for example, lemongrass (*Cymbopogon citratus*) essential oil has been shown to be effective against some strains of *Aspergillus* (Mishra & Dubey 1994). It is findings such as these, which could and should be used as the basis for clinical trials with the aim of reducing the quantity of some of the toxic and expensive drugs currently prescribed for fungal infections. It is hoped that through such work, ways can be found to incorporate essential oils into the clinical care of the haematology patient that are 'patient friendly', cheaper and as effective as the alternative super drugs. However, such innovations need to be carefully thought out and researched. Consequently, the author is currently working in collaboration with a scientist at Manchester University to move this work forwards.

In parallel with the research work above, the clinical service on the ALU has expanded and in some situations it is now integral to the medical care patients receive on the unit. By developing the service slowly and evaluating every step to ensure the safety and efficacy of the therapies offered, it has proved possible to offer massage to haematology patients undergoing active treatment. Equally, we have integrated these therapies into the patients' medical care, so greatly enhancing their quality of life through the work. It is both interesting and encouraging that the longer the service continues, more opportunities are opening up for using massage and aromatherapy in this setting.

INITIATING A MASSAGE SERVICE FOR HAEMATO-ONCOLOGY PATIENTS

For reasons which have been discussed previously, anyone wishing to start up a massage service in this setting is likely to encounter resistance. Therefore some recommendations for practical first steps in initiating such a service are given in Box 9.3.

SUMMARY

This chapter has described the difficulties faced by patients with haematological malignancies. Some of these difficulties have been illustrated by two case histories: The pathology of leukaemia has been discussed and recommendations have been made relating to setting up a service in the acute setting; The results of an audit of the service have been described together with some suggestions for future research and development of the service.

CREDIT

This chapter is based on an article published in Complementary Therapies in Nursing and Midwifery: Stringer J 2000 Massage and aromatherapy on a leukaemia unit, 6:72–76.

Box 9.3
Recommendations for setting up a service

- Therapists must have a good clinical understanding of haematological malignancies and their treatment.
- It is helpful to find a 'champion' – either a medical consultant or a senior nurse who supports the innovation.
- It is better to start with a small, safe and simple service that clinical staff feel comfortable with.
- All documentation should be in place before the project starts.
- It is important to think through the practicalities, e.g. 'Are facilities for blending essential oils and bases in a clinically clean environment available to the therapist?'.
- The multi-professional team may appreciate a presentation explaining the aims and objectives for the project. Feedback can be encouraged to gain insights from a different perspective.
- The project needs to be audited from the beginning to ensure that aims and objectives are being met. Audit also helps those involved to plan and implement the development of the service and also to learn from aspects of the project that did not work as well as anticipated.

REFERENCES

Cassileth BR, Vickers AJ 2004 Massage therapy for symptom control: outcome study at a major cancer centre. Journal of Pain and Symptom Management 28(3):244–249

Field T 2000 Touch therapy. Churchill Livingstone, London

Hayes J, Cox C 2000 Immediate effects of a five-minute foot massage on patients in critical care. Complementary Therapies in Nursing and Midwifery 6:9–13

Hernandez-Reif M, Ironson G, Field T et al 2004 Breast cancer patients have improved immune and neuroendocrine functions following massage therapy. Journal of Psychosomatic Research 57:45–52

Hoffbrand AV, Pettit JE, Moss PAH 2001 Essential haematology. Blackwell Science, Oxford

Mishra AK, Dubey NK 1994 Evaluation of some essential oils for their toxicity against fungi causing deterioration of stored food commodities. Applied and Environmental Microbiology 60:1101–1105

Post-White J, Kinney ME, Savik MS et al 2003 Therapeutic massage and healing touch improve symptoms in cancer. Integrative Cancer Therapies 2(4): 332–344

Seigel B 1986 Love, medicine and miracles. Harper & Row, New York

Tavares M 2003 National guidelines for the use of complementary therapies in supportive and palliative care. The Prince's Foundation for Integrated Health, London

FURTHER READING

Buckle J 2003 Clinical aromatherapy. Churchill Livingstone, New York

Cancer BACUP publications (www.cancerbacup.org.uk)

Macdonald G 1999 Medicine hands: massage therapy for people with cancer. Findhorn Press, Findhorn, UK

USEFUL ADDRESS

Jacqui Stringer
Clinical Lead Complementary Therapies
Christie Hospital
Wilmslow Road
Withington
Manchester M20 4BX
UK
Tel: 0161 446 3524

Collaborative working

10

Karen Livingstone and Anita Mehrez

Abstract

This chapter illustrates the benefits of a combined therapeutic approach in the management of symptoms of breast cancer treatment, bridging the best of conventional and complementary care. The origins and development of this approach will be described to illustrate how professionals can work together to provide a model service. The processes involved in this model, the collaboration between an aromatherapist and physiotherapist, will be discussed together with the perceived benefits of the service. Recommendations for maintenance and development of the service are given at the end of the chapter.

KEYWORDS

breast cancer, surgery, radiotherapy, mobility, body image, pain, exercise, touch, aromatherapy massage

INTRODUCTION

This unique collaborative project demonstrates good interprofessional working aimed at providing an integrated service for patients with cancer. The principles on which it is based reflect the recommendations of the National Institute for Health and Clinical Excellence (NICE) that complementary therapies need to be used, 'along side orthodox treatments with the aim of providing psychological and emotional support through relief of symptoms' (NICE 2004, p. 148). The model was developed in the Neil Cliffe Cancer Care Centre (described as the Centre hereafter) in the northwest of England. The centre is part of a larger hospice service (St Ann's) and serves as a multidisciplinary outpatient unit providing supportive care and rehabilitation to people with cancer and their families, within Manchester and the surrounding area. Patients from other acute cancer care services are able to self-refer to the Centre and a significant number of the service users have breast cancer. Access to the Centre may be at any point in the progression of the illness from diagnosis onwards.

At their first visit, patients receive a detailed assessment of their current physical, psychological, social and spiritual concerns with a key worker who is also a nurse. Following the assessment, patients are encouraged to set goals and a plan of action is negotiated. On completion of this process the patient is referred to the appropriate healthcare professionals within a multidisciplinary team. The key worker remains pivotal to co-ordinating and reviewing services for the individual patient.

One of the major aspects of work at the Centre is the physiotherapy service. A large proportion of breast cancer patients have a poor range of shoulder movements and associated pain and discomfort. Within this group there is a distinct subgroup with more complicated problems. These include reduced trunk mobility, fibrosis, abnormal adaptive posture pain and body image issues. The majority of patients are female as male breast cancer is one of the rarest malignancies (Borgen et al 1997). Patients who have post-surgical problems are referred to the physiotherapist who decides the best course of treatment. Where patients have more complex issues, such as those who are in the well-defined subgroup described above, they will usually be referred to the 'Symptom Control Clinic' for combined physiotherapy and aromatherapy.

The collaborative service evolved from the physiotherapist and aromatherapist liaising throughout separate courses of treatments for individual patients. It was decided to maximise the use of a combined approach where specialist physiotherapy and aromatherapy massage were used in the same clinic. The clinic became known as the Symptom Control Clinic (SCC), and its aim is to address the patient's physical and psychological problems in a dynamic and synergistic way which is giving excellent results.

COLLABORATIVE CLINIC ACTIVITY

Once the referral to the SCC has been made, the physiotherapist makes an assessment of the patient's problems, and discusses treatment aims. The patient attends the clinic for treatment at weekly intervals. To make the best use of time and the availability of rooms, and to facilitate the smooth running of the clinic, patients will first have some treatment from the physiotherapist. They then remain in the treatment room for a short time while the two practitioners consult and plan the follow-on aromatherapy massage. The aromatherapist treats the patient in the same room, thus saving the patient having to dress again and walk to another area. The physiotherapist then sees another patient in a second room and the aromatherapy treatment is again followed in the same room. This continual process ensures that the maximum number of patients can be seen in the clinic time. A combined appointment usually takes an hour and 20 minutes. The number of sessions allocated per patient is dependent on continual reassessment of progress. Liaison with the key worker is ongoing. This model of working facilitates inter-professional communication and allows for continuity of care for both patient and practitioners.

PROBLEMS ASSOCIATED WITH BREAST CANCER TREATMENT

Patients present at the clinic after one or more types of surgical intervention (see Box 10.1). In addition, they may have received other treatments such as radiotherapy, chemotherapy and hormone replacement. Presenting problems are many and varied. Their severity may depend on access to effective follow-up support, although there can often be a delay in this happening. Commonly, there is reduced range of movement, with pain and discomfort around the shoulder girdle, cervical spine and anterior chest wall, and there may be visible cording affecting extension at the elbow (Baum et al 1995, Downing 2001). After a course of radiotherapy there may be marked fibrosis and soft tissue tightness due to acute and chronic cell changes and occasionally neuropathic pain (DeVita et al 2001, Mohr et al 2001). Surgical breast reconstruction using latissimus dorsi or transverse rectus abdominis may lead to associated muscle weakness and muscle imbalance in the trunk. There can also be problems of recurrent swelling in the breast area and in the arm, i.e. lymphoedema. This may or may not have been addressed by a lymphoedema practitioner (see Chapter 12) and onward referral may be necessary. Overall, these patients will often present with poor posture and altered body image, a lack of confidence and a real fear of permanent disability (DeVita et al 2001).

BODY IMAGE ISSUES

It is likely that the experience of being diagnosed and treated for breast cancer will have had profound effects on a woman's life (Downing 2001, Neill et al 1998). By the time she comes to the symptom control clinic she will have followed through with a course of treatment which will have involved surgery and/or chemotherapy and radiotherapy involving numerous tests and investigations. She may be experiencing pain, stiffness, altered sensation and tightness, all of which remind her of the cancer and its effects on her body and emotions. She may also feel that this discomfort and/or pain has to be tolerated as the results of the cancer experience (see Case study 10.1). A reduction of symptoms such as pain and stiffness is important for the promotion of a

---

Box 10.1
Surgical interventions

- Simple lumpectomy or wide local incision with axillary node clearance
- Mastectomy and axillary node clearance
- Mastectomy, node clearance and immediate reconstruction, often a latissimus dorsi (LD) flap reconstruction, with or without implant
- Late reconstruction with tissue expanders and implant, LD flap or transverse rectus abdominis muscle (TRAM) flap, which is less commonly seen.

(Baum 1995, Downing 2001).

more positive body image. Often a limb that is painful and tight will feel bigger and be held protectively to the side, thus focusing the patient's attention on the treated area. The limb is no longer perceived to be able to function as normal and this perception hugely undermines her body image (Carver et al 1998). In the clinic, the physiotherapist aims to alleviate symptoms and teach and encourage regular home exercise. This approach helps to give the patient back a sense of control, thus promoting both improved function and independence. The addition of aromatherapy massage helps to enhance self-worth and release muscle tension, to improve sensation and to provide an enjoyable experience (Cawthorn & Carter 2000).

Case study 10.1

Two years previous to attending the SCC, Ann, aged 45 years, had undergone left mastectomy, chemotherapy and radiotherapy. Eighteen months later, she had LD flap reconstruction with a good cosmetic result. She reported feeling tightness in her trunk muscles and she was very aware of her abnormal posture. Ann did not know if this would improve and she occasionally wondered if she had done the right thing in having the reconstruction. After three treatments in the SCC Ann achieved full trunk mobility with improved posture, increased confidence in body image, improved sleeping pattern, and using Lavendula angustifolia (lavender) at home. Ann was delighted and surprised by her overall improvement in such a short time.

An experienced, compassionate and professional approach is needed to achieve successful management of body image concerns (Bredin 2001). Issues such as bra fitting, problems with prostheses, compression garments, and types of clothing, such as swimming costumes, can also be addressed. With the patient's consent, any unresolved issues or concerns raised within the treatment sessions are reviewed with the key worker. The concerns may be acted upon by other members of the multidisciplinary team, for example through accessing counselling or receiving nutritional advice from the dietician. Treatment may involve several sessions in the clinic and during this time the staff, through regular contact and discussion, will gain the trust of the patient, often giving emotional and practical support with issues such as bra fitting, problems with prostheses, compression garments and types of clothing such as swimming costumes.

THE PHYSIOTHERAPIST'S CONTRIBUTION

It is of vital importance that physiotherapists have oncology and palliative care experience and an in-depth knowledge of breast cancer and its treatments. They must work predominantly or exclusively with patients with cancer, and be able to provide expert advice and input for clearly defined rehabilitation needs (NICE 2004, p. 140). A detailed physical assessment of the body as a whole will identify structural and physiological impairment and enable the physiotherapist to create a treatment plan and to agree targets for improvement with the patient (Robinson 2000). Physiotherapy treatments usually include a wide range of progressive rehabilitation approaches involving exercise, stretches, mobilisations, and myofascial release techniques, combined with education about the body. The treatment will be based on an up-to-date awareness of the potential outcomes and complications of conventional cancer treatments. Strengthening of appropriate muscle groups with improved mobility and flexibility will supplement postural re-education and much work is done to improve overall appearance.

Patients are taught a system of regular home exercise to be done 'little and often' and this is reinforced with written instruction. This is because poor concentration and fatigue may be additional factors that need to be taken into account. Advice on lymphoedema and general skin care is given during the physiotherapy treatment and referral to a lymphoedema specialist is made when necessary. There will be feedback to the key worker and ongoing liaison with a wider team, such as the breast care nurse, surgeon and oncologist. It is important for specialist physiotherapists to access current literature and to networks and share practice development with others in the field (see Further reading and Useful addresses).

THE AROMATHERAPIST'S CONTRIBUTION

Aromatherapy treatment is usually given after the physiotherapy treatment so that patients leave the combined session feeling more relaxed through the release of tension, on a physical and emotional level. The aromatherapy massage also aims to improve the circulation in the muscle groups worked by the physiotherapist. The aromatherapist also reinforces the postural work which occurs throughout the symptom control treatment. Aromatherapy massage confers additional benefits when compared with non-aromatherapy massage (Fellows et al 2003, Wilkinson et al 1999). This therapeutic approach incorporates some powerful tools which promote relaxation. These include the stimulation of the sense of smell with an enjoyable aroma, and enable the patient to receive well-intentioned touch in the form of massage (Cawthorn & Carter 2000, Wilkinson et al 1999). Specific to breast cancer, Ritter (1999) found that women who have chest wall or arm pain as a result of scarring and cording after surgery, radiation therapy, or both, benefited from massage. Another long-term local complication is limited range of motion in the shoulder typically caused by pain, fear of movement and scarring. Ritter describes how massage and prolonged stretching often help to regain lose function and prevent further loss (see Chapter 3 for more detailed benefits of aromatherapy and massage). The SCC may be the first time that some patients have experienced aromatherapy massage and report feelings of relaxation, pleasure and perhaps acceptance of their cancer (see Case study 10.2). The references in Box 10.2 suggest positive indications for the use of aromatherapy massage pertinent to the SCC.

Case study 10.2

Sunita, aged 41, had a right mastectomy, chemotherapy, radiotherapy 2 years earlier. She presented in SCC following right reconstruction, prophylactic left mastectomy and insertion of tissue expander 4 months previously. When Sunita first saw the LD scar, she said she was 'more upset by the [LD] scar than by the first mastectomy'. Sunita presented with tightness in the right trunk, very tight rhomboids, and a marked reduction of her shoulder movement. Sunita's husband had to fasten her bra and she hated the sensation around the scar and on her right side.

During week 2, Sunita reported being able to receive massage around the scar area without feeling anxious and self-conscious. In week 3 Sunita was able to put on her bra herself and use a loofah on her back in the bath. At week 6 Sunita was discharged with: (i) full active range of movement in shoulder and trunk and good tissue extensibility; (ii) improved body image, and happier with the scar, she said, 'I have taken back my scar'; (iii) a relaxed posture; and (iv) much improved sleeping pattern.

Box 10.2
Examples of research work which supports the use of aromatherapy massage (see Chapter 3)

- Reducing pain intensity (Byass 1999, Field 1998)
- Altered body image following mastectomy (Bredin 1999)
- Inducing relaxation (Corner et al 1995, Diego et al 1998, Hadfield 2001)
- Reducing anxiety (Corner et al 1995, Shulman & Jones 1996, Wilkinson et al 1999)
- Improving wellbeing and quality of life (Wilkinson 1995)

Before there is any physical contact with the client, there is time for an initial consultation and feedback where anticipated outcomes are discussed and agreed. The massage starts with gentle holding through a towel to introduce the therapist's touch to the client. Muscles are relaxed with slow gentle effleurage movements to promote relaxation and to promote feelings of pleasure. It is important that any technique that causes pain or discomfort is avoided.

For patients who find it difficult to lie in a prone or a supine position, the use of a massage chair has been very useful. A patient can achieve an individual comfortable position. The arms, chest and head are fully supported and a comfortable position can be found for the back and legs. The chair can quickly and easily be 'fine tuned' to each client for optimum comfort, and access to the upper body is excellent, yet discreet (see Chapter 15). Supporting postural re-education and releasing the neck muscles during the massage is important so that the patient can feel the difference. Once the neck and shoulders are relaxed the patient may well be more able to notice physically how much longer her neck feels, how much lower her shoulders are, and how her overall posture has improved. Experiencing the massage and feeling a difference afterwards helps the patient to become more aware of when she has tension in her body, and when she is able to recognise it she can take some action to reduce it.

The two essential oils most often chosen by patients are *Rosa damascene* (rose) or *Lavendula angustifolia* (lavender). It is not within the scope of this chapter to go into detail about the essential oils used in the clinic but there is growing research to support the effects of individual essential oils (Buckle 2003). Individualised advice is also given to the patient about essential oils to use at home. This is supported by the provision of an introductory leaflet on aromatherapy, its uses and benefits. Continuing the use of essential oils is discussed prior to discharge. Patients are given more of their 'chosen blend' to use at home to help them replicate the state of relaxation. The use of the blend invites and facilitates gentle, physical contact with partners or those close to the patient. Applying the blend encourages the family to be involved in the patient's 'touch therapy'.

SUMMARY

In the service described in this chapter there is enhanced communication between the three members of the clinic, the patient, the physiotherapist and the aromatherapist. This ensures close co-operation to achieve the best possible outcome. Continual reassessment allows for rapid adaptability of treatment where necessary. Patients are highly compliant in their treatment continuing with both the exercises and the use of the aromatherapy blend to benefit the continuation of their treatments at home. The service allows patients to play a central role in their own recovery and rehabilitation, by 'taking an active role through self management' (NICE 2004, p. 135). The enthusiastic team approach gives motivation to both patient and other staff members within the wider multidisciplinary team. The team philosophy sees treating the person as a whole, rather than just working with an injured part as helping with nurturing patients who are often traumatised by their experience of conventional cancer treatments. The use of a joint physiotherapy and aromatherapy clinic ensures time and cost effectiveness for both the client and the centre with less overall visits and a seamless service. Additionally, the collaborative working and support assists individuals to boost their own body image and self-confidence. Suggested recommendations for developing similar services are listed in Box 10.3.

Box 10.3
Recommendations for collaborative working

Physiotherapists need to have:

● High level of skill and experience to treat patients with complications of cancer treatments.
● Opportunities to update their knowledge and skills.
● Managerial support and access to supervision to maintain and develop their work with patients.
● Professional contact with other healthcare professionals, e.g. oncologists, surgeons, breast care nurses, occupational therapists.

Aromatherapists/massage therapists need to have:

● Safe working knowledge of cancer treatments and related anatomy, including surgery techniques, radiotherapy, chemotherapy, complications and palliation.
● Information about developments in collaborative practice.
● Managerial support and access to supervision to maintain and develop their work with patients.

Shared responsibilities to:

● Acknowledge and appreciate each other's unique and skilled contribution to patient care.
● Maintain effective communication to enable a seamless service for patients.
● Audit, evaluation and research to maintain and develop the service.
● Disseminate best practice to encourage similar services to be available nationwide.

REFERENCES

Baum M, Breach NM, Shepherd JH 1995 Surgical palliation. In: Doyle D, Hanks GWC, MacDonald N (eds) Oxford Textbook of Palliative Medicine. Oxford University Press, Oxford

Borgen PI, Senie RT, McKinnin WMP et al 1997 Carcinoma of the male breast: Analysis of prognosis compared with matched female patients. Annals of Surgical Oncology 4:385–388

Bredin M 2001 Altered self-concept. In: Corner J, Bailey C (eds) Cancer nursing: care in context. Blackwell Science, Oxford

Bredin M 1999 Mastectomy, body image and therapeutic massage: a qualitative study of women's experience. Journal of Advanced Nursing 29(5): 1113–1120

Buckle J 2003 Clinical aromatherapy; essential oils in practice. Churchill Livingstone, London

Byass R 1999 Auditing complementary therapies in palliative care: the experience of the day-care massage service at Mount Edgcumbe Hospice. Complementary Therapies in Nursing and Midwifery 5:51–60

Carver A, Pozo-Kaderman C, Price A 1998 Concern about aspects of body image and adjustment to early stage breast cancer. Psychosomatic Medicine 60(2): 168–174

Cawthorn A, Carter A 2000 Aromatherapy and its application to cancer and palliative care. Complementary Therapies in Nursing and Midwifery 6(2): 83–86

Corner J, Cawley N, Hildebrand S 1995 An evaluation of the use of massage and essential oils on the well being of cancer patients. International Journal of Palliative Nursing 1(2):67–73

DeVita VT, Hellman S, Rosenberg SA 2001 Cancer: principles and practice of oncology, 6th edn, vols 1 and 2. Lippincott Williams & Wilkins, Philadelphia

Diego M, Jones NA, Field T et al 1998 Aromatherapy positively affects mood, EEG patterns of alertness and math computations. International Journal of Neuroscience 96:217–224

Downing J 2001 Surgery. In: Corner J, Bailey C (eds) Cancer nursing: care in context. Blackwell Science, Oxford

Fellowes D, Barnes K, Wilkinson S 2003 Aromatherapy and massage for symptom relief in patients with cancer. Complementary Therapies in Nursing and Midwifery 9(2):90–97

Field T 1998 Massage therapy effects. American Psychology 53(12): 1270–1281

Hadfield N 2001 The role of aromatherapy massage in reducing anxiety in patients with malignant brain tumours. International Journal of Palliative Nursing 7(6):279–285

Mohr KJ, Moynes Schwab DR, Tovin BJ 2001 Musculoskeletal pattern: impaired joint mobility, motor function, muscle performance, and range of motion associated with localized inflammation. In: Tovin BJ, Greenfield BHE (eds) Evaluation and treatment of the shoulder. FA Davis, Philadelphia

Neill KM, Armstrong N, Burnett CB 1998 Choosing reconstruction after mastectomy: a qualitative analysis. Oncology Nursing Forum 25(4):743–749

Ritter N, Love N, Osman D 1999 After breast cancer: implications for long-term primary care. Postgraduate Medicine 105(6):103–112

Robinson DJ 2000 The contribution of physiotherapy to palliative care. European Journal of Palliative Care 7(3):92–96

Shulman KR, Jones GE 1996 The effectiveness of massage therapy intervention on reducing anxiety in the work place. Journal of Applied Behavioral Science 32:160–173

The Prince's Foundation for Integrated Health and the National Council for Hospice and Specialist Palliative Care Services 2003 National guidelines for the use of complementary therapies in supportive and palliative care. London, The Prince's Foundation for Integrated Health and the National Council for Hospice and Specialist Palliative Care Services

Wilkinson S, Aldridge J, Salmon I et al 1999 An evaluation of aromatherapy massage in palliative care. Palliative Medicine 13(5):409–417

Wilkinson S 1995 Aromatherapy and massage in palliative care. International Journal of Palliative Nursing 1(1):21–30

FURTHER READING

Association of Chartered Physiotherapists in Oncology and Palliative Care 1993 Guidelines for good practice. Chartered Society of Physiotherapy, London

Chartered Society of Physiotherapy 2002 Standards of physiotherapy practice – core standards. Chartered Society of Physiotherapy, London

Chartered Society of Physiotherapy 2002 Rules of professional conduct, 2nd edn. Chartered Society of Physiotherapy, London

Clarke S 2002 Essential chemistry for safe aromatherapy. Harcourt Publishers, London

Constant C, Van Wersch A, Wiggers T et al 2000 Motivations, satisfaction and information of immediate breast reconstruction following mastectomy. Patient Education and Counselling 40:201–208

Tavares M 2003 National Guidelines for the Use of Complementary Therapies in Supportive and Palliative Care. The Prince's Foundation for Integrated Health and the National Council for Hospice and Specialist Palliative Care Services, London

USEFUL ADDRESSES

Association of Chartered Physiotherapists in Oncology and Palliative Care (ACPOPC)
Katherine Malhotra, Secretary of Membership
Physiotherapy Department
Royal Marsden Hospital
Fulham Road
London SW3 6JJ
UK
Website: www.acpopc.org.uk

Association of Physiotherapists Interested in Massage
Tessa Campbell
9 Woodfield Drive
Winchester
Hampshire SO22 5PY
UK

Karen Livingstone and Anita Mehrez
St Ann's Hospice
Neil Cliffe Cancer Care Centre
Wythenshawe Hospital
Southmoor Road
Wythenshawe
Manchester M23 9LT
UK
Tel: 0161 291 2912

11

Shiatsu for symptom management

Jill Bailey

Abstract

This chapter explains the origins of shiatsu and the principles on which it is based. The techniques used in shiatsu are explained in the context of traditional Chinese medicine and Zen shiatsu. Two case histories are used to illustrate the use of shiatsu in practice. Indications and contraindications are discussed and reference is made to traditional use of floor work and the merits of adapting treatments through the use of a massage chair. Insights into the way that shiatsu can be adapted are also explained. The chapter closes with a summary and recommendations.

KEYWORDS

shiatsu, traditional Chinese medicine, ki, meridians, tsubos shiatsu theory, yin and yang, elemental balance

INTRODUCTION

Shiatsu developed in Japan, although it originated in China over 2000 years ago. Its roots are in Chinese philosophy which originally had five components: acupuncture, medicines and herbs, the use of stones, moxibustion (the use of heat), and anma (massage). Shiatsu was developed from anma and over time it became anmo, which is the Japanese derivation. Shiatsu, as it is practised today, gradually evolved from anmo under influences from the East and the West. There are several styles of shiatsu, and the one which is most practised in the west is Zen shiatsu. This modern comprehensive system was created by Shizuto Masunaga who incorporated his knowledge of shiatsu into his knowledge of Western psychology and Chinese medicine.

A broad translation of the word 'shiatsu' is 'to apply pressure to the body using fingers' ('shi' means finger and 'atsu' means pressure). Shiatsu is applied by the use of the palms, the thumbs and the fingers. It can also involve sensitive and gentle stretching movements. Shiatsu is usually given through a thin layer of clothing, preferably in a natural fibre, with the patient lying on a futon (mattress) on the floor. An observer of shiatsu could easily perceive that it is a series of physical techniques. Gentle pressures are applied through the palms of the hand, and the therapist will seem to use different pressures in longitudinal directions both up and down the body. At times the therapist will use the thumbs or fingers to apply pressure locally.

THE CONCEPT OF KI AND THE MERIDIANS

Although the techniques are applied physically to the body, the aim of shiatsu is different from the aims of Swedish massage which is most often practised in the West. The aim of massage is to promote circulation through relaxing muscles and increasing the circulation. However, the aim of shiatsu is to re-balance ki (chi in Chinese). Ki can be described as the life force which flows everywhere through the body. This is not a concept that translates easily in the West; words like energy flow or 'life energy' are often used as the nearest translation. Ki is said to aggregate into channels where the flow is more concentrated; they run, like rivers, all over the body. These channels are called meridians and where one channel ends another begins. There are 12 major meridians and they connect with the major body organs and also functions of the mind and body. If the flow of ki in any part of a meridian becomes blocked, then flow of energy in another part of the meridian, quite separate from the part where the blockage is, may also be affected. The aim of shiatsu is to maintain health and vitality by ensuring that the flow of energy runs freely through all the organs and tissues.

THE NATURE AND ROLE OF TSUBOS

Along the meridians there are gateways or tsubos. These are pressure points where the ki can be accessed by the therapists 'needling' or pressing on a tsubo point. In shiatsu, ki is accessed by finger or thumb pressure as the whole length of the meridian is worked. (In acupuncture, ki is accessed through the use of very fine needles.)

THE PRINCIPLES OF SHIATSU DIAGNOSIS

The most common theories used by shiatsu practitioners in the West are those which underpin Zen shiatsu, traditional Chinese medicine and the Five Element Theory. The traditional methods used in shiatsu diagnosis are listening to the individual, observing physical and emotional characteristics, feeling by palpation and asking questions. The word diagnosis is not used in the same way as in Western medicine where the name of an illness or condition is sought before treatment can take place. Diagnosis in the Eastern sense is to take into account the results of the diagnostic procedure as described above and then the therapist uses some of the theories and techniques to rebalance the ki.

THE THEORY OF KYO AND JITSU

Jitsu means full and kyo means empty. In shiatsu, jitsu refers to where there is too much ki and kyo refers to where the energy in the meridian is depleted. Zen shiatsu diagnosis deals with the immediate state and energy distribution within the meridian network, so an understanding and application of these two concepts form an important part of shiatsu diagnosis and treatment. This is perceived in the initial diagnosis by palpation of either the hara or the back, which is usually carried out at the beginning of each session of shiatsu. The hara diagnostic area is an abdominal space which is bordered by the rib cage above, and below by the oblique lines from the anterior superior iliac spines and the pubic bone (Figure 11.1). All the meridians have a diagnostic area in the hara and palpation of this area reveals the most kyo and jitsu meridians. It is the information gained from the palpation of these two meridians which form the basis of the treatment session (see Figure 11.2). The back diagnostic area is used to diagnose more long-standing problems (see Figure 11.3).

THE KEY PRINCIPLES OF TRADITIONAL CHINESE MEDICINE

Life energy manifests itself in two opposing forces, yin and yang. These cannot exist without each other and must be in harmony for health. This principle of opposing and complementary forces was extended to include the five elements: wood, fire, earth, metal and water (Stevensen 1995). Early physicians believed that the cause and development of illness was based on the inter-relationship of these five elements and the way they influenced the flow of ki. Each organ in the body is related to an element and is either nourished or

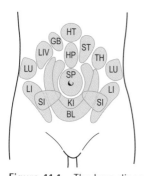
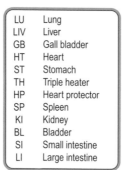

LU	Lung
LIV	Liver
GB	Gall bladder
HT	Heart
ST	Stomach
TH	Triple heater
HP	Heart protector
SP	Spleen
KI	Kidney
BL	Bladder
SI	Small intestine
LI	Large intestine

Figure 11.1   The hara diagnostic areas.

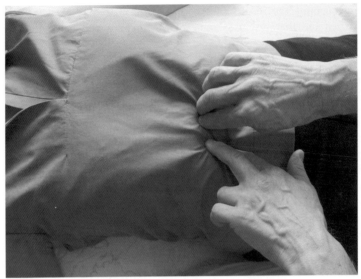

Figure 11.2   Hara diagnostic assessment of the abdomen.

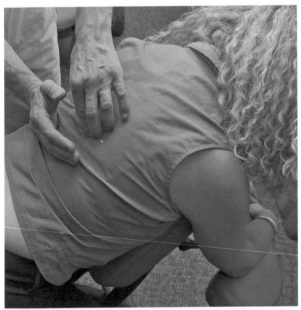

Figure 11.3   Hara diagnostic assessment of the back using the massage chair.

controlled by one of the other organs. Disease can be caused either by lack of nourishment or control of one organ by another as this imbalance interrupts the flow of ki. Traditional Chinese Medicine encompasses spiritual, emotional, mental and physical causes of disease, as well as taking into account factors such as diet, exercise and climate (Lundberg 1992). A brief explanation of

> ## Box 11.1
> ### An overview of the five elements used in traditional Chinese medicine and the related organs
>
> - Metal – lung and large intestine
>   This is associated with the emotion of grief, loss and the suppression of tears.
> - Wood element – liver, gall bladder
>   An imbalance is associated with inflexibility of tendons and psychological inflexibility, the emotion of anger and irritability. The liver energy rises and is concentrated in the head.
> - Fire element – pericardium and small intestine
>   Symptoms associated with the fire element are fevers, high temperatures, sweating, fear of heat, irritability and restlessness.
> - Water element – bladder and kidneys
>   The main symptoms are cold shivering pains in the joints, feeling chilled to the bone, with the accompanying emotion of fear.
> - Earth element – stomach and spleen
>   An imbalance of earth may manifest in the lower body and limbs, and present in feelings of heaviness, stiff swollen joints, tiredness and a dull heavy headache.
>
> Based on Lundberg (1992).

the properties and potential imbalances of the different elements is given in Box 11.1.

The elements are responsible for all aspects of human functioning and they comprise of ki, essence, blood, body fluids and the Shen or spirit. Shiatsu is a good treatment modality for the disharmonies of ki, in particular to aid the re-establishment of balanced ki flow throughout the body.

EASTERN DIAGNOSIS IN WESTERN PRACTICE

This methodology is not intended to replace Western diagnosis by a medical doctor. The word diagnosis could be interpreted as assessment of the individual's physical and emotional state, but in the context of shiatsu and its principles. In a Western context the sequence of events in a treatment could be as follows. When taking a history of the patient and the symptoms, the practitioner asks questions and listens for content of the response. He will also take notice of the patient's voice, appearance and demeanour, combined with her energetic and postural patterns when planning the treatment. Diagnosis is continued through palpation of the hara (or back). In some circumstances it may not be possible or appropriate to use hara or back diagnosis or to ask the patient questions. In this instance, a history could be obtained from medical staff and/or relatives. The treatment is then carried out. A treatment session usually lasts for an hour, but for a person who is frail and immunosuppressed, a session of 10 minutes' duration using gentle holding techniques to support the ki will be most effective. The hara or back is then reassessed and recommendations about self-help between treatments are given to the patient.

EFFECTS OF SHIATSU

In a nationwide study of the conditions which shiatsu practitioners treat, Harris and Pooley (1998) found that musculoskeletal and psychological problems were the commonest conditions with which individuals presented for shiatsu. These included, in particular, neck, shoulder and back problems; depression; and stress and anxiety. Cheesman et al (2001) carried out a quantitative study on patients attending a palliative care day service. On analysis, they found significant improvements in energy levels, improved relaxation, confidence, wellbeing and symptom control, clarity of thought and mobility. Bailey (1997) has published anecdotal articles on her work with people with cancer focusing on its important supportive role. The theories of shiatsu and traditional Chinese medicine are similar and therefore some of the research on acupuncture can be applied to the claims of shiatsu. For example a number of studies have shown that a point on the inside of the wrist, PC6, is more effective than placebo in reducing nausea in cancer chemotherapy (Dundee & Yang 1990, Price et al 1991). Some of the symptoms which have been found to respond well to shiatsu are listed below in Box 11.2. Case studies 11.1 and 11.2 illustrate how the principles and techniques of shiatsu are practised.

Box 11.2
Symptoms responsive to shiatsu in cancer and palliative care

- Stress, depression, anxiety
- Neck shoulder problems
- Back problems
- Fatigue and low energy
- Headaches
- Insomnia
- Pain
- Nausea
- Low self-esteem
- Feeling unwell and poor quality of life

Developed from Bailey (1997).

Case study 11.1

Mary, aged 55, had been diagnosed as having breast cancer 9 months previously. She had a right mastectomy and axillary node clearance followed by radiotherapy. Four months before presenting, Mary had experienced pain in her right shoulder and neck with a reduced range of movement, which was treated by a physiotherapist. The range of movement had increased, but the pain intensity and duration remained the same. Mary was referred for shiatsu by a nurse at a day centre for help with pain control and relaxation, although Mary was willing only to have shiatsu for pain relief.

PRESENTING SYMPTOMS

Mary's pain and reduction in movement in the right shoulder prevented her from doing daily activities including combing her hair and fastening her bra.

OBSERVATION

Mary's shoulders stooped and she held her right arm to her side. She had a rapid shallow breathing pattern and her voice had a whining complaining tone. Her face was whitish, and during the interview she was suppressing tears.

EXAMINATION

Subjective

Mary described herself as doing well to get over the cancer and regaining control of her life, although she found the pain and restricted movement debilitating.

Objective

Mary was not able to comply with a hara diagnosis as she felt that palpation of the abdomen would be intrusive.

Energy pattern

The therapist observed that there was a weakness in the ki in the upper chest and a concentration of ki in the head.

Local palpation of the meridians

On assessment the lung meridian in the arm was kyo (empty). The liver meridian was jitsu, or full, in the head and neck.

TREATMENT

Aims

1. *Tone the lung meridian in the arms, chest and throat.*
2. *Bring the energy down towards the legs to encourage flow in the throat and arms.*
3. *Use dispersing techniques for the liver and gall bladder meridians, particularly in the shoulders and neck.*

Home treatment

Over the course of the treatments, Mary was taught how to perform self-shiatsu or do-in exercises for the lung and liver meridians, together with breathing exercises to promote the flow of lung ki. Shiatsu sessions were agreed at weekly intervals for 3 weeks. Following a review three more sessions at weekly intervals were given.

Session 1

Focus was only on the shoulders, neck and right arm as Mary wished these areas to be treated. Afterwards, Mary reported a reduction in pain intensity although she was unable to relax during the 2-minute session.

Session 2

Mary allowed the hara diagnosis and accepted treatment to the whole body over 30 minutes. She reported a reduction in pain and felt relaxed during the session. While receiving shiatsu to the lung meridian in the arm she verbalised her sadness and sense of loss. There was a change in the distribution of ki in the body observed and felt by the shiatsu practitioner. The pain relief lasted for 2 days, but when the pain returned it was less intense.

Sessions 3–6

Pain was now at a manageable level and Mary was able to fasten her bra and comb her hair without discomfort. The lung and liver energies were more balanced, the concentration of ki in the head had dispersed and the energy in the chest area was stronger. This was demonstrated by Mary's improved posture, pinker complexion and steadiness of breath.

Case study 11.2

Yvonne, aged 33, was supporting her mother who had been diagnosed as having lung cancer. Unable to relax or sleep she sought help from the palliative day care service. Yvonne was struggling with both a full-time job and supporting her mother, with whom she had an ongoing difficult relationship.

EXAMINATION

Subjective

Yvonne described experiencing tension in the muscles of her neck, shoulders and back, fatigue and poor sleep pattern. Recently, she had also developed mouth ulcers.

Objective

Throughout the assessment Yvonne continued to smile and put on a brave face in contrast with the difficult problems she was describing.

Energy pattern

Her energy, or ki, was concentrated around the neck and shoulders with a weakness of ki in the legs and lower back.

Hara diagnosis

Her small intestine meridian was jitsu (excess ki) and bladder was kyo (empty ki).

Local palpation of the meridians

The small intestine meridian was jitsu in the neck and shoulders, and the bladder meridian was kyo in the legs and lower back.

ANALYSIS

There was an imbalance in the small intestine meridian, which is closely linked with the other meridians in the fire element, i.e. heart (associated with the assimilation of physical and emotional changes). An imbalance could produce blood stagnation in the abdomen and tension in the neck and shoulders. Mouth ulcers are also associated with a concentration of ki in the head and neck. The bladder is linked with the water element and a kyo condition produces a lack of impetus and low back pain.

AIMS OF TREATMENT

1. *Tone the bladder meridian and so reduce the jitsu in the small intestine meridian.*
2. *Bring the energy down from the neck and shoulders and encourage the flow of ki reducing any stagnation.*

TREATMENT

Yvonne had a course of five sessions, fitting them in with her work and caring commitments. The sessions initially lasted 20 minutes, as she was unable to rest for any longer. By the last two sessions she was able to receive treatment for 40 minutes. Initially, Yvonne described an increased feeling of relaxation and well-being. By the end of session 5 she was able to relax and not feel restless. Her level of fatigue, and neck, shoulder and back pain had reduced. She had been able to talk with her mother about some of the long-term issues that had caused difficulties in their relationship. On observation, the upper body and lower body energy levels were more balanced.

WORKING WITH CARERS

As an important step in integrating shiatsu in cancer care, it could be offered to carers and staff (see Case study 11.2). Formby (1997) has established a shiatsu service for carers of older patients.

CONTRAINDICATIONS TO SHIATSU

It would be unwise to give shiatsu when some conditions are present although some adaptations can be made. As shiatsu works directly over the body the contraindications are similar to those for general massage. Some contraindications have been suggested by Stevensen (1995); these are common to other massage and bodywork (see Box 11.3). Importantly, an experienced therapist can adapt the intervention safely in certain circumstances, such as where there is difficulty receiving touch. The patient can be treated over clothes or through a towel, with a choice to stop the treatment at any point (see Case study 11.1).

ISSUES FOR THE SHIATSU PRACTITIONER

Positioning using a futon or massage chair

Using a futon allows versatility for the shiatsu practitioner to use hands, elbows, knees and feet and a variety of stretches and allows them to adopt a good posture. People also feel comfortable, relaxed and supported receiving shiatsu when lying on a futon. Some people, however, may be unable to get

---

Box 11.3
Suggested contraindications to shiatsu

- Difficulties in receiving touch
- Osteoporosis, fractures, bony metastasis
- Burns, wounds, broken skin or infectious diseases
- Unexplained swellings or any new pain in the area to be treated
- Lymphoedematous limbs
- Over operation sites for 1–2 months
- Directly over varicose veins
- Tendency to bruising or over present bruising
- Pyrexia
- Clotting dysfunction
- Directly to the area receiving radiotherapy

Stevensen (1995).

down and up from the floor. There also may not be enough space for a futon and the room may be draughty at floor level, for example in a ward environment. The shiatsu practitioner may also be unable to work from the futon due to knee problems. Alternatives include working from an ordinary chair, a treatment couch, bed or a massage chair. In addition the techniques can be adapted (see Figure 11.3). Table 11.1 compares the advantages and disadvantages of the futon and massage chair.

Table 11.1
Comparison of the use of the futon and massage chair

	Futon	Massage chair
Advantages	The futon can be rolled up and moved depending on its size	Portable and quick to set up in small space, e.g. ward area or small room
	The position is secure and comfortable for the person to receive a full treatment	Avoids wear and tear of therapist's knees and back and the therapist can still maintain an open posture
	The therapist can access all of the patient's body	Good position to apply techniques to back, arms, shoulders, neck
	Hara and back diagnostic areas can be accessed easily	Can use back diagnostic area People report it as a comfortable position
Disadvantages	The patient may have difficulty in getting on and off the floor	Comfortable for a 15–20-minute treatment session
	Lying on the futon may be uncomfortable in a draughty or cold, i.e. uncarpeted, room	Cannot access chest area and parts of leg or use hara diagnostic area
	Risk of wear and tear of the knees of the shiatsu practitioner	

Adaptations and managing responses to treatment

In practice, there are few side effects when the timing, positioning and techniques of shiatsu are adapted to the person's needs. However, there may be an initial aggravation of symptoms after the treatment. Should this happen, the length of the treatment may be reduced or the frequency of the treatments decreased. Alternatively, a lighter touch may be required. Following a treatment, a patient may feel sleepy and very relaxed. Although this can be a positive experience, this may not be desired if the patient has to travel. The next treatment can be modified as has previously been described. These possible responses highlight the need to be guided by the person's needs and wishes. Shiatsu therapists need to assess and regularly review the treatment plan, and liaise with the patient's multidisciplinary team. In working with people who are affected by cancer, a guiding principle is to cautiously build up the length of treatments and the depth of touch.

SUMMARY

While popular in a community setting, shiatsu has yet to be fully integrated in cancer care. There is a paucity of research and published case work. Part of the difficulty is there is only a small, but growing, number of therapists working in this specialty. Recommendations for developing integrative shiatsu in cancer care are given in Box 11.4. This chapter, written by an experienced physiotherapist, has given an overview of shiatsu and its adaptation to cancer care. The essence of shiatsu is gentle work on the body's soft tissues with a deep-acting effect, making it a safe body therapy in the management of symptoms. Although the chapter has focused on patients, the intervention would also be of benefit in improving the wellbeing of carers.

Box 11.4
Recommendations

- Practitioners must be experienced and understand the physical and emotional aspects of working with people with cancer.
- Make adaptations for patients with symptoms, such as fatigue and immobility, for example by working in the chair.
- A useful starting point for promoting the use of shiatsu is offering treatments to carers and staff.
- Shiatsu therapists need to ensure that patients have sufficient understanding of the therapy, the techniques used and the benefits and responses before engaging in the treatment.
- Healthcare professionals require knowledge and understanding of the practice to inform patients and make appropriate referrals.
- There is a need for quality research work about the benefits and safety of shiatsu in cancer care.

REFERENCES

Bailey T 1997 Shiatsu and cancer – a personal reflection. Shiatsu Society News 62:16–17

Cheesman S, Christian R, Cresswell J 2001 Exploring the value of Shiatsu in palliative care day services. International Journal of Palliative Nursing 17(5):234–239

Dundee JW, Yang J 1990 Prolongation of the anti-emetic action of P6 acupuncture by acupressure in patients having cancer chemotherapy. Journal of the Royal Society of Medicine 83:360–362

Formby J 1997 Shiatsu massage for carers. Complementary Therapies in Medicine 5:47–48

Harris PE, Pooley N 1998 What do shiatsu practitioners treat? A nationwide survey. Complementary Therapies in Medicine 6:234–239

Lundberg P 1992 The book of shiatsu: vitality and health through the art of touch. Gaia Books, London

Price H, Lewith G, Williams C 1991 Acupressure as an antiemetic in cancer chemotherapy. Complementary Medicine Research 5:93–94

Stevensen C 1995 Shiatsu. In: Rankin-Box D (ed) The nurse's handbook of complementary therapies. Churchill Livingstone, London

FURTHER READING

Batterman A 2000 Shiatsu with physiotherapy and integrative approach. In: Charman RA (ed) Complementary therapy for physical therapists. Butterworth-Heinemann, Oxford

Beresford-Cooke C 1996 Shiatsu theory and practice. A comprehensive text for the student and professional. Churchill Livingstone, Edinburgh

Hammer L 1990 Dragon rises red bird flies. Station Hill Press, New York

Jarmey C 1991 Shiatsu foundation course. Godfield Press, Hampshire

Kaptchuk TJ 1991 The web that has no weaver, 6th edn. Ryder, London

Macioca G 1980 The foundations of Chinese medicine. A comprehensive text for acupuncturists and herbalists. Churchill Livingstone, Edinburgh

Ridolphi R, Franzen S 1996 Shiatsu for women. Harper Collins, London

USEFUL ADDRESS

The Shiatsu Society UK
Eastlands Court
St Peters Road
Rugby
Warwickshire CV21 3QP
UK
Tel: 0845 1304560
Email: admin@shiatsu.org.
Website: www.shiatsu.org

Managing lymphoedema

12

Cheryl White

Abstract

This chapter gives a brief overview of lymphoedema and some guidance for complementary therapists on how to approach a treatment when a patient presents with chronic oedema. The aim is to increase understanding of the nature of the condition, and to establish an awareness of the complexity of lymphoedema treatments. Optimising patient care through collaborative working is discussed and key issues for the massage therapist, including contraindications and ways of adapting massage treatments, are described. Recommendations for therapists are included.

KEYWORDS

lymphoedema, causes and treatment, infection, complementary therapy, key issues, collaborative working

INTRODUCTION

Lymphoedema is a complex, chronic and often debilitating condition, characterised by the swelling of a body part. The swelling results from the failure of the lymphatic drainage system with an associated accumulation of protein-rich fluid in the soft tissues (British Lymphology Society 2001, Jeffs 1993, Mortimer 1990). The extremities are usually affected, although the swelling may be found in the adjacent area of the body such as the face, head, neck, trunk or genitalia. Lymphoedema is usually unilateral in distribution but it can be bilateral. There is no cure for the oedema; the aims of treatment are to reduce the swelling or prevent it from worsening, and to restore limb shape and prevent associated complications, such as infection (Mortimer 1997). The psychological morbidity and psychosocial problems, which often occur in patients with lymphoedema, are addressed in treatment programmes in order to improve a patient's overall quality of life (Woods 1993).

ROLE OF THE LYMPHATIC SYSTEM

The lymphatic system is a one-way drainage system which has an important part to play in maintaining a steady balance of fluid within the body. The system transports a colourless fluid known as lymph around the body from the tissues to the blood vascular system. Lymph is primarily made of protein and water. The protein particles are large and move back into the capillaries slowly and with difficulty. Lymphatic vessels are much more permeable than blood vessels and have a role in picking up the proteins and returning them back to the circulation (Badger 1996, Mortimer 1990). The lymphatic system also transports some hormones, enzymes, fat and waste products, and has a role to play in the body's defence mechanism against bacteria and mutant cells.

The lymphatic system has a superficial network of vessels known as the initial lymphatics which lie just under the surface of the skin and in all soft tissues. Fluid and waste products are collected from the four regions of the body known as quadrants (Figure 12.1). These feed into a deeper network of vessels and, after being filtered by the lymph nodes, lymph fluid returns to the circulation via two large lymphatic trunks in the chest known as ducts. These then drain into the large veins at the base of the neck (Casley-Smith & Casley-Smith 1997).

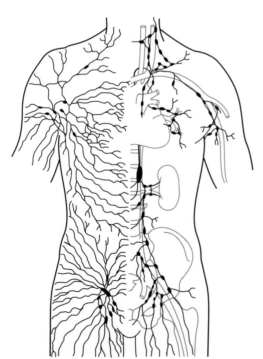

Figure 12.1   Distribution of the lymphatic system in the four quadrants of the body.

By stimulating the lymphatic system with certain treatment modalities, it is possible to move fluid from one quadrant of the body to another, passing over dividing boundaries known as 'watersheds'. If the deeper vessels are blocked the more able areas of the system work harder and assist with the drainage (Foldi et al 1985).

PRIMARY AND SECONDARY LYMPHOEDEMA

Lymphoedema is classified as primary and secondary. Primary lymphoedema is due to a mechanical insufficiency of the lymphatic system. There is an intrinsic defect of the lymphatic pathways, and it is a congenital or hereditary condition, e.g. Milroy's disease (Browse et al 2003). Secondary lymphoedema usually has a known cause, an extrinsic factor that damages the lymphatic system anatomically. This can be due, for example, to trauma, burns or infection. In patients with cancer, the disease or its treatment (e.g. surgery or radiotherapy) can cause obstruction or a disturbance in the lymphatic and venous systems (Mortimer 1995). When the oedema has been caused solely by the failure of the lymphatic system, this is termed 'true' lymphoedema. Other chronic oedemas, such as lymphovenous oedema, result from various other peripheral causes such as venous insufficiency, poor venous return and limb immobility. In patients who have cancer, oedema can be present with or without the presence of active disease.

It is thought that once the axillary lymph nodes have been removed or damaged during surgery or radiotherapy, the lymph vessels fail to regenerate and the function of the lymphatic system at this point in the body is compromised. Irradiated, scarred tissue decreases the transport capacity of the lymphatic system. This results in accumulation of high-protein fluid in the tissues (Mortimer 1990).

STAGES IN THE DEVELOPMENT OF LYMPHOEDEMA

The initial stages of lymphoedema are described in Box 12.1.

Box 12.1
Initial stages in the development of lymphoedema

1. Fluid accumulates in the tissues and may be noticed as swelling. Initially this may be slight and the tissues remain soft and may 'pit' on palpation.
2. There may be a feeling of tightness or tension. The patient may describe the limb as feeling heavy.
3. Initially the swelling is of an even distribution and will be limited to one limb.
4. There may be a pink tinge to the skin which may surmount to being described as inflammation.

In the early stages, the condition is relatively easy to treat. However, it is often ignored or dismissed as being an acceptable level of oedema, especially if it is not interfering with function (Jeffs 1993, Mortimer 1990). If treatment is not forthcoming, the swelling may increase, and the distribution may take on an uneven appearance and extend to adjacent areas, such as the trunk and genitalia.

The accumulation of protein-rich fluid in the skin and tissues leads to characteristic changes in the skin. Dry skin indicates that there are excess proteins in the tissues drawing necessary moisture from the skin, and the presence of hyperkeratosis indicates that the protein has been stagnant for some time. The skin loses its elasticity and papillomatoses, small blisters, can form (Mortimer 1990, Veitch 1993). The subcutaneous tissues become fibrotic and feel thickened when touched, and skin folds may appear deepened or enhanced. Stemmer's sign, which is the inability to pick up skin at the base of the second digit, is often positive and differentiates lymphoedema from other types of swelling (Casley-Smith 1992, Mortimer 1995).

RECOGNISING LYMPHOEDEMA

Early diagnosis and treatment of lymphoedema is important, but often difficult. The oedema may not appear immediately after cancer treatment, but may develop many months or even years later (Figure 12.2). Patients should be educated about minimising the risks of developing the condition, advised on the signs and symptoms, and where to access assistance should they develop any oedema in the future. All healthcare professionals should be aware of the symptoms, as they are likely to come into contact with patients at risk of, or who already have, lymphoedema. If the patient is not already having treat-

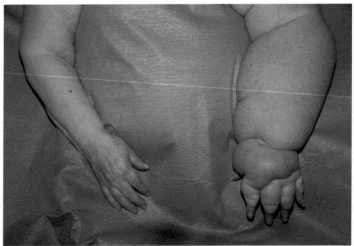

Figure 12.2 Secondary lymphoedema of the arm. (Photograph by Katrina Moore, Christie Hospital NHS Trust, Manchester, UK.)

ment, referral to the local lymphoedema service should be made because if left untreated it is likely to get worse (Casley-Smith 1992).

Before treatment for lymphoedema commences, a detailed assessment of the patient is undertaken by a lymphoedema specialist. The medical history is obtained by referring to the medical notes and from interviewing the patient. Patients are asked about the development of the swelling and the factors that influence an increase or reduction, and also about the effects of any previous treatment. Clinical observations include an examination of the skin and sub-cutaneous tissues. The circulation is assessed and if the lower limb is involved, a Doppler ultrasound reading may be undertaken (International Society of Lymphology 1995). The degree and distribution of the swelling are assessed and detailed measurements are taken as an objective record (Stanton et al 1996). Patients are questioned about any functional difficulties they may have and a basic psychological assessment is undertaken to help gauge motivation and their likely response to treatment. The treatment will have to become part of a patient's daily life and he or she needs to be willing to take responsibility for the long-term management of the condition. The aim is to offer patients assessment, education and support, helping them to cope with and manage their own care as far as possible (Cameron & Gregor 1987). Having completed the assessment, a patient's condition can be rated according to the four cat-egories listed in Box 12.2.

PROBLEMS FACED BY PATIENTS WITH LYMPHOEDEMA

Physically, patients with lymphoedema may present with a multitude of func-tional difficulties which need to be addressed. A patient with lower limb oedema may become less mobile as the oedema may restrict the distance he can walk or the use of stairs may be difficult. As a patient's limbs become more dependent, the muscle pump in the legs is not stimulated and the lym-phatic system comes under more strain. Patients with arm oedema may not

---

Box 12.2
Categories of lymphoedema

Patients do not remain static in each group but will move between the categories depending on their response to treatment and on their disease process.

- People 'at risk' of developing lymphoedema
- People with mild and uncomplicated oedema
- People with moderate, severe or complicated oedema
- People with oedema and advanced malignancy

British Lymphology Society (2001).

be able to hold a pen, write, or use cutlery correctly. Fine movements can be severely affected if the hand is swollen and the individual may be more prone to accidents in the home.

The integrity of the skin is compromised, and taut and dry skin is easily damaged. A simple knock may result in a skin break and possible infection. Patients who have lymphoedema are already vulnerable to episodes of infection in the skin known as cellulitis as it is felt that the immune system itself may be compromised. The poor movement of lymph inhibits the infection fighting mechanisms and serves as an excellent medium for the development of bacterial and fungal infections. Cellulitis can cause fever, malaise and a red, inflamed, tender limb thus making the patient very unwell. It needs to be treated immediately with antibiotics and sometimes requires hospitalisation (Jeffs 1993).

Psychosocial effects of having lymphoedema also vary, and it is felt that the degree of swelling does not necessarily correlate with the level of psychological distress. Even the smallest amount of oedema can cause an individual a significant degree of stress (Woods 1993). It is accepted that patients who present with breast cancer-related swelling experience increased psychosocial maladjustment and psychological morbidity with regard to their disease, when compared with those who do not have any swelling (Woods et al 1995). Both the condition and the treatment can have a stigmatising effect. Emotionally, the person may already have an altered body image due to the extent of the surgery, and a swollen limb may add to the problem. The swelling and the use of compression garments may leave a patient feeling different from other members of society, acting as a constant reminder of the disease and the treatment she has experienced. Some may become depressed and isolated and this may interfere with relationships. They may be conscious about the reaction of others, which may inhibit socialising. Patients may show anger and resentment at the situation especially if the oedema presents well after their initial diagnosis or when treatment has been completed. Practically, patients may not be able to wear their chosen style of clothing, and if the feet are swollen, may find it difficult to buy footwear that either fits or looks acceptable. For some, this may lead to a loss of interest in appearance and a loss of self-esteem (Tobin et al 1993, Woods 1995). Social activities such as sport, walking or even shopping can become restricted or impossible for some; this can have an immense impact on a patient's morale. Employment may be affected, especially if the person has a very physical or highly skilled job. Alternative employment can be limited (Badger 1996) depending on the site and extent of the lymphoedema.

TREATMENT OF LYMPHOEDEMA

The principles behind the physical treatment of lymphoedema rely on interventions that enhance the lymph flow and maximise any remaining lymph transport capacity. The ultimate aim is to remove excess protein from the tissues (Foldi et al 1985). However, successful management will be influenced by the underlying cause of the oedema and how long the swelling has been established. Treatment also addresses factors such as immobility, poor function or infection, which will inhibit lymphatic flow further and possibly exacerbate existing oedema (Mortimer 1990). Discomfort and pain are not normally associated with lymphoedema, although the patient may describe an ache or feeling of heaviness and tightness. Specific areas of pain need to be investigated further by medical staff (Badger 1996). The four elements of lymphoedema treatment are stated in Box 12.3.

Skin care

Meticulous skin care is of paramount importance in the treatment of lymphoedema (Jeffs 1993), the aim being to prevent infection and hydrate the skin, thus maintaining suppleness. The presence of the protein-rich fluid in the tissues is an ideal environment for bacteria to grow, and by maintaining the integrity of the skin the risk of infection is limited. Patients are encouraged to follow a daily skincare routine, taking care to dry the skin carefully and gently after washing, and to apply moisturiser to their limb. They are advised to clean any areas of broken skin thoroughly, to apply antiseptic cream and encouraged to avoid sunburn, insect bites and cuts (Mortimer 1990, Regard et al 1991).

Exercise and movement

Exercise utilises muscular activity to compress the lymphatic vessels and the surrounding tissues. This in turn promotes lymph flow and enhances the uptake of fluid via collateral drainage routes. Exercise also has a positive effect on joint movement and function. Patients are encouraged to undertake a daily exercise programme, which consists of exercises or movements specific to their problems, age and the site of the oedema. Any activity or exercise should be performed at a steady rate, which stimulates lymph flow, rather than excessive, strenuous activity, which is thought to stimulate arterial blood flow and may

---

Box 12.3
The cornerstones of lymphoedema treatment

All four of the following factors are used in combination to achieve the maximum benefit for the patient:

- Skin care
- Exercise and movement
- Lymphatic drainage
- External support

have an undesired effect on the oedema (Badger 1996). The benefits of exercise are accelerated if external compression garments are worn during exercise. Although it is important to intersperse periods of rest while exercising, complete immobility of the limb is discouraged as this suppresses muscular activity (Mortimer 1997). Activities such as walking and swimming are also encouraged as good all-round exercises.

Specific massage for lymphoedema

Patients are taught simple lymphatic drainage (SLD), a form of lymphatic massage, which uses a series of gentle hand movements on the skin. The slow, rhythmical movements are performed in the direction of the lymph flow towards the nearest functioning set of regional lymph nodes. Lymph is encouraged to move from swollen, congested areas, via the skin and superficial lymphatic vessels, to areas where it can drain more easily. The technique is based on the principles of manual lymphatic drainage (MLD), which is performed by the therapist. It initially concentrates massage on the normal lymph draining areas such as the opposite side of the body and the trunk. Once drained, these areas are able to accept fluid from the swollen limb more readily (Foldi et al 1985).

External support

External support is given to the limb using garments such as arm sleeves and hosiery or multilayer lymphoedema bandaging (MLLB). The exerted pressure encourages the fluid to drain from the limb by enhancing the muscle pump and increasing the uptake of the lymphatic system. It also limits the formation of lymph (Badger 1996, Mortimer 1990). Each form of support has a distinct purpose and is used at a specific stage of treatment. Bandages are used to reduce oedema and restore the limb's normal shape, whereas hosiery is designed to support the tissues once they have been drained to maintain the shape and size of the limb (Badger 1996). Due to the high compression pressures required to treat lymphoedema, both the application of bandages and the assessment and provision of compression garments should be undertaken by a lymphoedema specialist with the appropriate knowledge, skills and training.

Long-term management consists of maintenance treatment which aims to conserve the shape of the limb and condition of the skin. Once patients have been taught by the lymphoedema specialist, they engage in daily self-management, which consists of skin care, exercise, simple lymphatic drainage, and if prescribed, the use of external compression garments. This is coupled with regular monitoring and support from the lymphoedema specialist. If the oedema does not respond to this package of care, or if there is an increase in severity or added complications, a course of intensive treatment may be necessary. This consists of skin care, exercise, MLD and MLLB, and it is undertaken by the lymphoedema specialist. The aim is to reduce the size of the limb, and to restore or maintain the integrity of the skin and tissues. The regimen is followed on a daily basis for 2–4 weeks, and is given alongside the maintenance treatment.

All treatment requires commitment and perseverance by the patient. A long-term, daily routine can be time consuming and tiring, and often requires necessary adjustments to an individual's lifestyle. In chronic illness, the outcome of a treatment programme depends on the patient's ability to maintain the regimen, although this is difficult when there is no envisaged cure (Cameron & Gregor 1987). Non-compliance is one of the most common reasons for deterioration in the state of a limb.

KEY ISSUES FOR COMPLEMENTARY THERAPISTS

Lymphoedema is not necessarily a contraindication for some complementary therapies, but cautions and considerations must be adhered to, to avoid further deterioration in this condition. Ideally, the massage therapist should work alongside the lymphoedema specialist, so that the patient gains the maximum benefit from both treatments (Tavares 2003). Collaboration between service providers and therapists enables co-operation and a mutual sharing of skills and knowledge, reinforcing the shared aim of enhancing the patient's quality of life (Howells & Maher 1998). See Chapter 10 on Collaborative working for further discussion of multidisciplinary working.

First, complementary therapists should be aware of the patient's illness and consider what problems may be encountered (Filshie 2001). Before working with a patient with lymphoedema the medical notes must be accessed, or at least an accurate and up-to-date account of the patient's condition obtained from nursing or medical staff. It will be helpful if the massage therapist knows if the patient has advanced or progressive disease, and whether or not he or she is in pain. It is vital that the therapist is aware of complications such as deep vein thrombosis. For all of these scenarios, treatment must be adapted and, on occasions, it may even be contraindicated in its entirety. Second, massage therapists need to consider whether there is any risk that they could cause a patient more harm than good, especially if treating a patient with any conditions outside their scope of practice and expertise (see Chapter 4). Therapists can also refer to organisational policies and procedures where a patient's symptoms are particularly complex (Tavares 2003). Once these issues have been carefully considered and resolved the massage therapist, in consultation with the lymphoedema specialist, can work safely with the patient, setting realistic goals in relation to the proposed intervention.

PRACTICE POINTS

It is essential the patient is comfortable and cushions or pillows are used to support heavy swollen limbs. The affected area may be gently elevated to just above the heart level, if this can be tolerated by the patient (Mortimer 1995).

If the therapist is using massage it is important to work with the physiology of the lymph system, so the therapist massages away from the swollen area towards the unaffected side. Gentle touch is important and passive movements are useful where the therapist is able to help a patient move the limb. If a patient is capable of moving, they can be encouraged to do some gentle exercise (under the guidance of a lymphoedema specialist), which may even initiate a slight increase in the lymphatic drainage (Mortimer 1997). Movements used with a swollen limb should be slow and methodical in nature as heavy or repetitive movements may worsen the condition. All therapists should treat the limb or swollen area with respect.

Therapists should consider the link between the development of lymph-oedema and tissue trauma and possible infection. Patients are advised not to have any form of venepuncture or injections in the affected limb or in a limb that is at risk of developing lymphoedema (Jeffs 1993). Since broken skin is a source of potential infection, the avoidance of acupuncture in this area is also advised (Filshie 2001). Acupuncture carries the potential risk of infection due to the invasiveness of the needles (Shen & Glaspy 2001) and instances of cellulitis following acupuncture in an oedematous limb have been reported (White et al 2001). Recommendations therefore include the avoidance of needling an oedematous area with selection of an alternative site, where possible (Filshie 2001).

All therapists should always wash their hands prior to treating a patient and be mindful of any fragile skin or cuts. Breaks in the skin can become infected easily and may increase the oedema (Jeffs 1993). Such areas should be cleaned and antiseptic cream applied in order to limit the possibility of contamination. Therapists are advised not to treat over any areas of infection or cellulitis. Clearly massage in this area would be uncomfortable, and there may also be the added risk of spreading infection via the lymphatic system (Jeffs 1993). Cellulitis can make patients feel very unwell and they require immediate medical advice and antibiotics. The suspension of any lymphoedema treatment is advised with the emphasis on rest and elevation of the limb (Jeffs 1993). Patients are also advised to apply emollients or cream to their limb or swollen area daily to maintain the skin's moisture and prevent dry areas. Specific skin problems should be treated with the appropriate dermatological treatments (Williams & Venables 1996). Aromatherapists should be aware of the fragility of the skin and consider this when selecting oils and creams (Tavares 2003). Research work on the benefits of essential oils and bases with lymphoedema is required before any recommendations can be made.

It is important to avoid deep pressure over lymphoedematous areas. The importance of gentle pressure is paramount as the function of the superficial lymphatic vessels can be restricted with heavy touch. Deep massage to any area of the body should be avoided in a patient who has active cancer in order to avoid trauma and activation of the immune response (Tavares 2003). The already compromised drainage may be affected further and the oedema worsened (Casley-Smith & Casley-Smith 1997). Similarly, treatments which involve acupressure or aromatherapy massage need to be approached with caution. All therapists need to understand why the patient may have an area of oedema. If, for example, a patient's abdomen is oedematous, they may have ascites. If this is the case massage should be avoided over this area (Tavares 2003).

Reflexology can be performed on patients with lymphoedema, although this may be difficult if the feet are swollen. When the reflexologist is unable to work on the feet, the patient's hands can provide a useful alternative. Therapists can work in conjunction with a lymphoedema specialist if they are unsure if the area should be avoided (Tavares 2003), see Chapter 14.

The overall physical and psychological state of the patient needs to be considered; some will have undergone extensive surgery and treatments and may have a swollen limb to add to their difficulties. The patient may have body image issues and may not wish to expose a particular body area. In this case, the massage treatment should be adapted to meet the needs of the patient. Even when massage is given for a short length of time, the treatment can be beneficial both psychologically and physically (see Case study 12.1).

Case study 12.1

Mary, aged 42, was receiving inpatient palliative radiotherapy for advanced breast cancer. Her dominant (right) arm was grossly oedematous with little movement, and her daily living activities were affected. Mary was advised about using moisturising cream and encouraged to use the unaffected arm to assist with some movement in her right arm. She was shown how to position the arm on a pillow for support and to maintain slight elevation using a soft sling. Mary was also offered palliative bandaging to the limb to help control the oedema and give it some support, which she accepted. In addition to her physical symptoms, Mary experienced low-self esteem and body image problems.

Mary requested some massage for relaxation and it was agreed that reflexology and foot massage would be the most appropriate approach. Mary received her treatments while sitting in a chair with her legs supported on a stool. This position helped her to breathe more easily. The use of positive touch and massage by the lymphoedema specialist and the reflexologist assisted Mary to feel more comfortable as well as helping her to cope with treatments for her long-term illness.

SUMMARY

Many patients present with oedema but it is important to remember that not all limb swelling is lymphoedema. This condition can be chronic and debilitating requiring a thorough assessment and detailed treatment planning. Management is specialised and long-term, requiring a high degree of self-management and commitment from the patient. Complementary therapies are not necessarily contraindicated but if alternative treatment areas are inaccessible the opposite side of the body or another limb may receive some gentle work. Therapists need to be sensitive to the patient's problems and diagnosis, access medical notes or seek confirmation that therapies are appropriate and not contraindicated. Additional care and awareness is essential with this group of patients in order to avoid an exacerbation of the condition. Close liaison with the local lymphoedema specialist is fundamental to optimise treatment for the patient and produces valuable, collaborative working between the two services. Recommendations for safe and informed practice are listed in Box 12.4.

Box 12.4
Key recommendations

To work safely therapists are advised to:

- Collaborate with the multi-professional team to ensure a seamless and safe service.
- Have a working knowledge of lymphoedema, including the anatomy and physiology of the lymph system, its causes, treatments and complications.
- Recognise boundaries of practice, e.g. therapists should not carry out any diagnosis or interventionist treatment, or give advice on managing lymphoedema. (This is the role of lymphoedema specialist.)
- Attend study days tutored by a lymphoedema specialist to update knowledge.
- Be aware of body image issues and effects of treatment on social, physical and psychological wellbeing.
- Seek advice immediately from a lymphoedema specialist or appropriate healthcare professional if there are changes in the oedema and/or reddening of the skin.
- Adapt treatments to avoid any trauma to oedematous tissues, e.g. with reflexology, unaffected hands may be worked rather than an oedematous foot.

ACKNOWLEDGEMENT

The author thanks Justine Whitaker, Clinical Nurse Specialist, Lymphoedema, East Lancashire, for proofreading the chapter.

REFERENCES

Badger C 1996 The management of lymphoedema In: Denton S (ed) The management of lymphoedema in breast cancer nursing. Chapman and Hall, London, pp. 204–215

British Lymphology Society 2001 Chronic oedema population and needs. British Lymphology Society, Sevenoaks

Browse N, Burnand KG, Mortimer PS 2003 Diseases of the lymphatics. Hodder Education, London

Cameron K, Gregor F 1987 Chronic illness and compliance. Journal of Advanced Nursing 12:671–676

Casley-Smith JR, Casley-Smith JR 1997 Modern treatment for lymphoedema, 5th edn. Bowden Printing, Adelaide

Filshie J 2001 Safety aspects of acupuncture in palliative care. Acupuncture in Medicine 19(2):117–122

Foldi E, Foldi M, Weissleder H 1985 Conservative treatment of lymphoedema of the limbs. Angiology 36:171–180

Howells N, Maher EJ 1998 Complementary therapists and cancer patient care: developing a regional network to promote cooperation, collaboration, education and patient choice. European Journal of Cancer Care 7:129–134

International Society of Lymphology Executive Committee Consensus Document 1995 The diagnosis and treatment of peripheral lymphoedema. Lymphology 28:113–117

Jeffs E 1993 The effect of acute inflammatory episodes (cellulitis) on the treatment of lymphoedema. Journal of Tissue Viability 3(2):51–55

Mortimer PS 1990 Investigation and management of lymphoedema. Vascular Medicine Review 1:1–20

Mortimer PS 1995 Managing lymphoedema. Clinical and Experimental Dermatology 20:98–106

Mortimer PS 1997 Therapy approaches for lymphoedema. Angiology 48(1):87–91

Regard C, Badger C, Mortimer PS 1991 Lymphoedema advice on treatment, 2nd edn. Beaconsfield Publishers, Beaconsfield

Shen J, Glaspy J 2001 Acupuncture: evidence and implications for cancer supportive care. Cancer Practice 9(3):147–150

Stanton AWB, Levick JR, Mortimer PS 1996 Current puzzles presented by post mastectomy oedema (breast cancer related lymphoedema). Vascular Medicine 1:213–225

Tavares M 2003 National guidelines for the use of complementary therapies in supportive care. The Prince's Foundation for Integrated Health, London

Tobin MB, Lacey JH, Meyer L et al 1993 The psychological morbidity of breast cancer related arm swelling – psychological morbidity of lymphoedema. Cancer 72(11):3248–3252

Veitch J 1993 Skin problems in lymphoedema. Wound Management 4:42–45

White A, Hayhoe S, Hart A et al 2001 Survey of adverse effects following acupuncture (SAFA): A prospective study of 32,000 consultations. Acupuncture in Medicine 19(2):84–92

Williams AE, Venables J 1996 The management of skin problems in uncomplicated lymphoedema. Journal of Wound Care 5:223–226

Woods M 1993 Patients' perceptions of breast cancer related lymphoedema. European Journal of Cancer Care 2:125–128

Woods M 1995 Sociological factors and psychosocial implications of lymph-oedema. International Journal of Palliative Nursing 1(1):17–20

Woods M, Tobin M, Mortimer PS 1995 The psychosocial morbidity of breast cancer patients with lymphoedema. Cancer Nursing 18(6):467–471

FURTHER READING

Foldi M, Foldi E, Kubik S (eds) 2003 Textbook of lymphology for physicians and lymphedema therapists. Urban & Fischer, San Francisco, CA

Mortimer PS, Badger C, Hall JG 1998 Lymphoedema. In: Doyle D, Hanks GWC, Macdonald N (eds) Oxford Textbook of Palliative Medicine. Oxford University Press, Oxford, pp. 657–665

Twycross R, Jenns K, Todd J (eds) 2000 Lymphoedema. Radcliffe Medical Press, Oxford

USEFUL ADDRESSES

British Lymphology Society (BLS)
PO Box 196
Shoreham
Sevenoaks
Kent TN13 9BF
Tel: 01959 525524
Website: www.lymphoedema.org/bls

Lymphoedema Support Network (LSN)
St Luke's Crypt
Sydney Street
London SW3 6NH
Tel: 020 7351 0990
Website: www.lymphoedema.org/lsn

MLD[UK]
PO Box 14491
Glenrothes
Fife FY6 3YE
Scotland
Tel/fax: 01592 748008
Website: www.mlduk.org.uk

Massage and spinal cord compression

13

June Rosen and Joanne Carr

Abstract

The project described in this chapter developed in response to a request for patients to have foot massage. As patients with spinal cord compression (SCC) often present with reduced distal sensation a major concern for therapists is not doing any harm. The service was initiated from a partnership between two physiotherapists, with one working as a complementary therapist. The chapter starts by describing the condition of SCC, its symptoms and treatments, and continues with the development of the project through a planned audit. Case studies are included to illustrate the value of this carefully managed intervention.

KEYWORDS

spinal cord compression, SCC, care pathway, massage, physiotherapy and teamwork

INTRODUCTION

The spinal cord is the part of the central nervous system that runs through a narrow canal protected by numerous vertebral bodies. Spinal cord compression (SCC) is a devastating presentation of metastatic malignant disease. It occurs when the contents of the dural sac, the spinal cord or the cauda equina become damaged as a result of compression by a tumour mass or a collapsed vertebra that has been replaced by bone metastases. It is an extremely complex and challenging condition for health professionals, and SCC is considered an oncological emergency requiring prompt investigation and treatment.

Referrals to treat patients with SCC have increased since complementary therapies became more widely available at the project site. Patients have reported that massage has helped with altered sensation, temperature and mobility. As this was anecdotal, and treatments such as radiotherapy, steroids and physiotherapy are usually in place, it is important that the contribution of massage be evaluated.

SIGNS AND SYMPTOMS

The minimum radiological evidence for SCC is indentation at the level corresponding to the clinical findings, which can include any or all of the following: local or radicular pain (pain experienced in a dermatome due to root pressure), weakness, sensory disturbance and/or evidence of sphincter dysfunction (Loblaw & Laperriere 1998). SCC occurs in up to 5% of patients, and it is a devastating complication of cancer both for the patients and their carers (Doyle et al 1998). At-risk primary sites for SCC and areas affected are listed in Box 13.1. Patients may experience severe pain and discomfort in the lower limbs, and may also present with changes in muscle tone. Spasticity and increased tone can cause painful involuntary movements and stiffness, whereas decreased tone results in limbs feeling heavy and cumbersome. Altered sensitivity can add to the patient's discomfort, with a range of strange feelings from complete numbness to increased sensation. There can be pain on even the lightest of touch – this is termed 'allodynia' and is used to describe pain caused by stimulus that does not normally provoke pain (Haller et al 2003).

Box 13.1
'At-risk' primary sites for SCC and spinal areas affected

Primary cancer sites

- Lung – 16–19%
- Breast – 12–13%
- Prostate – 7–18%
- Others:
  - Kidney
  - Melanoma
  - Sarcoma
  - Multiple myeloma
  - Thyroid
  - Gastrointestinal

Spinal areas affected

- 10% affect the cervical region – mainly breast
- 70% affect the thoracic region – mainly lung and breast
- 20% affect the lumbosacral region – gastrointestinal and prostate tumours, melanoma

---

Sources: Chen (2001), Downing (2001), Falk & Fallon (1997).

The earliest symptom of SCC is back pain, which may have been present for weeks or months prior to the compression. Patients often describe a 'tight band-like pain', which can be aggravated by coughing, sneezing or movement. It may radiate around the trunk and down into the lower legs (Downing 2001). Patients can sometimes 'pinpoint' the origins of the pain in a defined area of back, which usually coincides with the level of the compression. Medical advice can be delayed if early symptoms are confused with muscle strain or existing degenerative joint disease. Analgesic medication may have been used with little relief. Muscle weakness in the presence of back pain may have hastened a patient's referral for investigation. The onset can be rapid, varying from slight foot drop to inability to weight bear, which can be both catastrophic and frightening for the patient. The weakness may be symmetrical or asymmetrical, relative to the level of the cord compression and the corresponding motor distribution. Altered sensation below the level of compression is another key symptom, although not always present. The autonomic control of the bladder and bowels is often compromised and patients may be distressed by urinary retention, constipation or complete loss of bladder and bowel control. It is only when a complete picture of the patient's history, signs and symptoms are considered together that a diagnosis of SCC can be made. 'Red flag' symptoms of SCC are listed in Box 13.2.

INVESTIGATIONS

A clinical history is required including signs, symptoms, duration and any possible triggering events. For example, a fall may have led to a vertebral fracture in a patient with bony metastases. A neurological examination should include

---

Box 13.2
Red flag symptoms of SCC

If a patient has a known history of cancer the following symptoms need prompt medical advice/investigation to exclude SCC:

- Intermittent and/or progressive back pain.
- Exacerbation of an existing back related problem.
- Any recent injury/strain that results in pain and/or alteration in sensation in any extremities.
- Report of a tight band or restriction related to level of back pain.
- Report of recent localised back pain.
- Increased use of/unresponsive to, analgesia for back pain.
- Altered sensation in the extremities described as tingling, cotton wool, painful to normal touch, numb, heavy, etc.
- Muscle weakness at the level or below the site of back pain.
- Altered bladder and/or bowel function.

muscle and sensation testing together with upper and lower motor neurone testing. Proprioception testing needs to be done as this loss is usually indicative of poor neurological recovery. Plain radiological films may reveal SCC from bone destruction, but not all compressions are detectable. A magnetic resonance imaging (MRI) scan is therefore the investigation of choice (Cook et al 1998). A whole spine scan will show where there is more than one level of compression. All evidence suggests that the later the presentation the bleaker the outcome in terms of function and prognosis (Solberg & Bremnes 1999). In the most severe cases it may mean that a patient becomes completely paraplegic, wheelchair dependent and needing continual help.

STABILITY OF SPINE

The concern for SCC management is the stability of the spine, i.e. whether or not movement is safe without risk of further compression. In the case of suspected SCC instability should be assumed until clinical features and/or radiological imaging suggests otherwise. For example, a scan may indicate vertebral collapse, where one vertebra has slipped forward onto another. Pain, triggered by movement, may be indicative of spinal instability. Movement, for example, of a limb, may also result in sensory changes, e.g. patient reporting 'pins and needles', or any kind of 'shooting' or 'electric shock-like' sensations.

REHABILITATION PROGRAMME

Physiotherapists have specialist training in motor system assessment, with their early input adding to the overall clinical assessment and treatment. A baseline measure of tone, power and sensation is performed against which progression or deterioration can be monitored. In the early stages the patient may need to be immobilised to prevent further damage to the spinal cord. This will involve flat bed rest and care as if they had an acute spinal injury, e.g. log rolling to manoeuvre the patient. For a cervical compression a hard collar may be fitted to immobilise the patient's neck. Again the physiotherapist can advise on handling issues and the fitting of the collar. Patients are given advice and exercises to maintain circulation and prevent respiratory complications. Apart from medical treatment (usually radiotherapy and steroids) occupational therapists and other members of the multidisciplinary team are involved to achieve maximum function for the patient (Lablow & Laperriere 1998). At all stages of rehabilitation, realistic goals need to be set with patients, as sadly some do not recover movement or function.

The risks of prolonged bed rest have to be balanced against those of movement causing further damage. A bedside assessment of spinal instability is essential, including how leg movements, either active or assisted, and gentle rolling in the bed affect symptoms. If symptoms are aggravated, the physiotherapist may decide to proceed with caution or to return the patient to a flat position and discuss analgesia with the multidisciplinary team. If gentle bed movements cause no symptom aggravation, the patient may be moved into a semi-recumbent position. Once the patient is able to sit at 90°, it may be possible to take the legs over the side of the bed and to be in full sitting. This activity allows an assessment of truncal tone and balance to be made. Progressing onto standing is dependent on the power in the lower limb muscles and the ability to maintain an unsupported seated position. The physiotherapist will provide an individualised exercise programme to re-educate and strengthen weak muscles. Transfer from bed may require a variety of moving and handling equipment and training.

BACKGROUND

Until the SCC and massage project began only hand massage or relaxation techniques were offered to patients. One particular patient was insistent that she received a foot massage. Prior to providing the treatments the therapist met with the physiotherapist to decide how best to proceed. The therapist was struck by the comment that the patient felt 'more complete' after the treatment, and that although she had limited sensation, it was 'good to have attention to my feet' (see Case study 13.1). A structured project was proposed with the aim of exploring the possibility of providing safe and adapted foot massage for people with SCC.

Case study 13.1

Agnes, aged 76, developed SCC after a primary carcinoma of the lung. Her skin was very dry and papery. Agnes had no sensation to touch although she reported that her right leg felt slightly colder. There were some involuntary foot movements. She had massage to her feet and lower legs, which she enjoyed. She said that it made her feel pampered – a new experience – and requested further treatments. Agnes's skin became supple and she repeated how much she valued 'being pampered'. Both she and her daughter stated how helpful the treatment had been, particularly as it had been given to the part of her body that 'didn't work', which meant that she no longer felt 'incomplete'.

It was decided to monitor the frequency of referral and treatment, with a massage protocol designed in collaboration with a physiotherapist (see Appendix 13.1). When planning the project the team considered asking patients to complete a questionnaire, but given the severity of their condition it was felt it would be an inappropriate burden. A decision was then made to conduct an audit to monitor the frequency of referral, type of cancer, number of treatments and the verbal feedback from the patient. An important element of the service was the ongoing collaboration between the specialist physiotherapist and the massage therapists.

Clinical audit involves the systematic review of processes, procedures and services used for diagnosis, care and treatment of patients in the clinical setting. It usually examines how resources are used and reports on the effect that care has on the outcome and quality of life for the service users (Department of Health 1996). Audit can be the first stage in a formal evaluation study or research project to investigate clinical work and provide information that might be of value to patients, clinicians and service providers, locally or nationally (see Chapter 3).

A total of 36 patients with confirmed diagnosis of SCC were referred to the project but 28 (13 males and 15 females) were treated. A further 12 patients were referred with unconfirmed diagnosis of SCC and were also treated using the massage protocol. Reasons for non-treatment included: too ill (n = 3), transferred to a hospice on the day of referral (n = 4) and death (n = 1). The number of treatments ranged from one to five sessions, with patients receiving an average of three treatments during their hospital stay. A sample of treatment data over a period of 2 months is shown in Table 13.1. It is important to note both positive and negative feedback. However, all patients treated were grateful and appreciative of the intervention, and requested that the treatment be continued (see Table 13.1 for examples of comments). It does need to be acknowledged that this feedback was given to the therapist who provided the treatment. As patients with SCC can experience variability and/or deterioration in their condition, it is important for the therapist to consult with either the physiotherapist or the medical team prior to each treatment session (see Appendix 13.1). Given the severity of the patient's illness relatives often wished to be present, and besides appreciating the time and attention given, found it relaxing just to watch (see Case studies 13.2 and 13.3). It is recommended that the outcomes for this intervention should be formally evaluated, with data collected by researchers not involved in providing the treatments (see Case study 13.3).

Case study 13.2

Diane, aged 45 years, had metastases in the spine secondary to breast cancer. On returning to the ward after a trip to the garden, the nurse noticed that her feet were cold and cyanosed, which she herself had not noticed. She wore nothing on her feet and they were not supported on the footplates of her wheelchair. A concern raised by the therapist was the possibility of injury, due to Diane's diminished sensation. She was offered a foot massage and experienced a feeling of warmth in her feet after the treatment. The therapist advised her to wear socks that did not give any constriction and for her feet to be raised and supported comfortably when sitting.

Table 13.1
A sample of spinal cord compression treatment details

Name	Gender	Age (years)	Cancer	Massage sessions	Compression area/concerns/observations	Patients' post-treatment comments
Ken	Male	45	Testicular	3	Areas of pain: Lumbar 3/4 Numbness and discomfort in lower limbs, loss of mobility and very anxious	First session: 'More sensation in left leg. Much more comfortable and relaxed' Second session: 'I have been looking forward to this all day' Third session: 'More please'
Noel	Male	47	Forearm sarcoma	2	Compression at Thoracic 2 Loss of mobility and diminished sensation in lower limbs Urinary catheter in place	First session: 'More sensation and feel very relaxed' Second session: 'Much more comfortable and warmer'
Jim	Male	33	Hodgkin's lymphoma	2	Area of pain: Thoracic 6/7 Formerly a footballer Awaiting liver stent Mobilising with physiotherapy – but finding it very difficult because of reduced sensation in lower limbs, 'my legs feel like cotton wool'	First session: 'So pleased to have treatment, very relieved to have some sensations – so grateful' Second session, partner was present, reporting: 'I felt relaxed just watching – I'm glad something is being done that helps'

Table 13.1 continued over

Table 13.1
A sample of spinal cord compression treatment details—cont'd

Name	Gender	Age (years)	Cancer	Massage sessions	Compression area/concerns/observations	Patients' post-treatment comments
Sandra	Female	50	Spine	4	Destruction of Lumbar 4 vertebra Diminished sensation in lower limbs and anxiety	First session: 'Much more comfortable – floaty and relaxed' Third session: 'I could have this for hours'
Sheila	Female	55	Breast	1	Compression noted at Thoracic 7/8 Heavy legs, uncomfortable and restricted mobility Altered sensation in hands – 'can't pick up a pen' Pain on elevation of legs	'Enjoyed the sensation, feet felt more comfortable'

Case study 13.3

Ron, aged 62 years, had been active and working. He had been diagnosed with renal carcinoma after presenting with a short history of a cough and back pain. Soon after Ron had complained of increased back pain and difficulty in walking. A scan revealed SCC at the level of Thoracic 8/9. His pain was controlled by analgesia via a syringe driver. He only had movement in the middle two toes of his right foot. He also had a past history of depression. Ron was given massage to his feet and lower legs; this provided comfort but also allowed him the much-needed opportunity to go over the events of his illness. Ron repeatedly spoke of the illness as a great loss, a kind of bereavement. He spoke of not being able to drive or go upstairs – these things were clearly important to him.

Ron's wife and son were present during his treatments, which allowed a relaxed time for sharing family experiences, and even to laugh. He had deteriorated but was hoping to be transferred to the local hospice. Ron gained a degree of acceptance, with his family finding the treatments to be comforting and helpful. They valued that 'something beneficial could be done' for someone for whom 'nothing could be done'.

Box 13.3
Recommendations/concerns for SCC massage practice

- Massage therapists should be aware of SCC and its symptoms.
- Any 'red flag' symptoms should prompt a therapist to recommend the patient with a history of cancer to seek medical advice/further investigations.
- Ensure the patient is assessed prior to treatment and consents to treatment.
- Work by a massage therapist must be in collaboration with physiotherapist and the multidisciplinary team.
- Any changes in sensation in the affected limbs must be recorded, ideally using the patient's own words.
- The relative's wish to stay during treatments, with agreement of patients, must be appreciated.
- Where there are changes in sensation the therapist is required to use gentle pressure, while being mindful of the altered sensation.
- Attention to limbs with reduced functions and sensation may lead to patients sharing their worries and concerns.
- There is a need to conduct research in this area, to formally evaluate and disseminate outcomes for this intervention.

SUMMARY

Given the complexity of the patient with SCC condition and likely poor prognosis, identifying interventions that bring comfort and relaxation is important to helping patients cope emotionally. Many of the patients in the audit were relatively young with rapid disease progression. A massage service needs to operate in close collaboration with the patient's physiotherapist as well as the rest of the multidisciplinary team. Given that patients can have both pain and numbness, massage must be adapted with careful monitoring of their responses, and as with any other medical conditions, if in doubt do not treat. In these circumstances the therapist may want to consider offering a non-touch relaxation technique, such as guided imagery. A summary of recommendations and concerns are listed in Box 13.3.

Appendix 13.1
Massage and SCC audit activity

The standard to be audited

Patient with either new or enduring spinal cord compression will be offered a minimum of two 20-minute complementary therapy treatments per week as part of an integrated SCC care pathway.

Recent provision

An informal review of the complementary therapy service identified that treatments were appreciated by patients with SCC. The principal referrers were physiotherapists. Experience of providing this service has identified the need for complementary therapists and physiotherapists to collaborate so that an efficient, safe and integrated service is ensured. It is proposed that the service is delivered and audited to inform and evaluate the standard proposed.

Aims of the audit

- To monitor referral rates, access and uptake of the service
- Gather data to inform structure, process and outcomes of the service standard

Intervention

Treatment will be given using a massage protocol adhered to by all therapists and monitored by the project leader. Two sessions will be offered per week.

Data to be collected

- Referral date
- Referrer

- Location, age, gender, diagnosis, level of SCC
- Sensory assessment performed by senior physiotherapists
- Date of first treatment and frequency of treatment
- Feedback from patient

Massage protocol for patients with SCC

Massage is given to the feet and lower legs, aiming to complete the treatment of both feet within 20 minutes. Additionally, at the end of the session a 5-minute relaxation technique can be offered.

Therapist preparation

- Physiotherapy referral and medical agreement to offer massage.
- Treatments are to be given by audit team members only, qualified both as a healthcare practitioner (nurse or physiotherapist) and a massage therapist.
- Therapists must adhere to handwashing hygiene as required by the hospital/Trust policy.
- An adjustable swivel chair on wheels is recommended for the therapist's comfort.
- Ensure informed consent (information about the treatment and project, with the emphasis on patient choice to receive or not and the right to stop the massage treatment at any point).
- Discuss optimal and safe positioning of patient prior to treatment with physiotherapist.
- Assess and note areas of increased or diminished sensitivity and any allodynia.

Patient preparation

- Support of limbs, if in sitting, legs need to be elevated to 90% hip flexion with pillow support under knee.
- Calves free of any restriction.
- Remove thrombo-embolism prevention stockings and splints and replace at the end of the session.
- Time: 20 minutes.

Massage technique

- Medium – grape seed oil (skin tested).
- Establish contact – holding the feet gently but firmly to create contact, mindful of areas with changes in sensation.
- Note the degree of tension and holding, temperature and condition of skin, nails and circulation.
- Effleurage strokes from the feet over lower legs and up to knees.

- Supporting the limb with one hand, work the opposite side of the calf and then reverse to work the other side.
- Use circular movements to massage around the malleoli.
- Support the foot with one hand and massage the dorsum of the foot using short effleurage strokes, followed by intra-tendon work using the fingers.
- Hold the dorsum of the foot and knead the plantar surface.
- Thumb strokes up the sole, followed by massage to each toe in turn.
- Complete the treatment by effleurage to the lower limb, followed by gentle downward strokes and holding for a few moments.

Passive movements

Care must be taken not to exceed the normal range of movement. The following movements can be integrated into the session on advice from the physiotherapist. These include:

- Plantar flexion and dorsiflexion.
- Inversion and eversion.
- Ankle rotation in both directions.
- Individual toe rotation and gentle extension.

Work each foot separately monitoring patient's response and after holding the foot for a few moments repeat the sequence on the other foot. Each movement should be done three times. Enclose the feet and lower limbs in a towel. A short imagery and/or relaxation technique can be included.

REFERENCES

Chen TC 2001 Prostate cancer and spinal cord compression. Oncology 15(7): 841–855

Cook AM, Lau TM, Tomlinson NJ et al 1998 Magnetic Resonance Imaging of the whole spine in suspected malignant spinal cord compression: impact on management. Clinical Oncology 10(1):39–43

Department of Health 1996 Using clinical audit in the NHS: a position statement. NHS Executive, Leeds

Downing J 2001 Acute events in cancer care. In: Corner J, Bailey C (eds) Cancer nursing: care in context. Blackwell Science, Oxford

Doyle D, Hanks GW, MacDonald N (eds) 1998 The Oxford Textbook of Palliative Medicine, 2nd edn. Oxford University Press, Oxford

Falk S, Fallon M 1997 ABC of palliative car: emergencies. British Medical Journal 315:1525–1528

Haller H, Leblhuber F, Trenkler J et al 2003 Treatment of chronic neuropathic pain after traumatic central cervical cord lesion with gabapentin. Journal of Neural Transmission 110(9):977–981

Loblaw DA, Laperriere NJ 1998 Emergency treatment of malignant extradural spinal cord compression: an evidence-based guideline summary. Journal of Clinical Oncology 16(4):1613–1624

Solberg A, Bremnes RM 1999 Metastatic spinal cord compression: diagnostic delay, treatment, and outcome. Anticancer Research 19:677–684

FURTHER READING

Corner J, Bailey C (eds) 2000 Cancer nursing: care in context. Blackwell Science, Oxford

Higginson I (ed) 1995 Clinical audit in palliative care. Radcliffe Medical Press, Oxford

USEFUL ADDRESS

Joanne Carr and June Rosen
C/o Rehabilitation Unit
Christie Hospital NHS Trust
Wilmslow Road
Manchester M20 4BX
UK

14

Creative approaches to reflexology

Edwina Hodkinson, Barbara Cook and Peter A Mackereth

Abstract

Reflexology as a therapy is becoming increasingly popular in many countries. In the UK the therapy is commonly available in hospices for both patients and their carers. There has been some reticence about using reflexology in acute cancer care settings, especially when patients are receiving conventional treatments such as radiotherapy and/or chemotherapy. This chapter reviews the theories and practice of reflexology, clarifies concerns and then describes innovative approaches to safely adapt treatments for patients and the carers in cancer care settings.

KEYWORDS

reflexology, concerns, adaptations and innovative approaches

INTRODUCTION

The use of reflexology in cancer care is becoming popular and is widely offered in the UK within most hospices, specialist cancer centres and oncology units (Graham 1998, Kohn 1999). Reflexology is also becoming more accepted by healthcare professionals as a valuable way of helping patients to manage the stresses and anxieties that accompany the cancer journey (Hodkinson & Williams 2002). Providing reflexology to patients diagnosed with cancer can create challenges for the therapist, both professionally and personally. First, students of reflexology may have been told that the intervention is contra-indicated, without any evidence to support this statement. Second, patients living with cancer and its treatments may be too fatigued to tolerate an hour-long session. Third, complications and disease progression (e.g. spinal cord compression), as well as essential conventional treatments, such as chemo-therapy, radiotherapy, steroids and analgesics, may influence perceived sensation and skin integrity (see Chapter 13). When assessing the appropriateness of offering a patient reflexology it is essential that the therapist consults with the wider healthcare team. Adapting the intervention to the individual ensures that the therapy is used both gently and safely.

ORIGINS, THEORIES AND PRACTICE OF REFLEXOLOGY

The practice of reflexology is believed to have originated in China over 5000 years ago. There is also pictorial evidence of the feet being worked for health benefits in Egyptian and North American Indian art (Griffiths 1996). In the early twentieth century Dr Fitzgerald, an American laryngologist, began investigating and writing about the theory and practice of reflexology, renaming it 'reflex zone' therapy. Later, in the 1930s, Eunice Ingham, a nurse and physiotherapist, developed detailed maps of the feet. Ingham is considered to be the 'matriarch' of Western reflexology, having been responsible for established training for health professionals and lay practitioners. Doreen Bayley trained with Ingham and is accredited with establishing the first of many British reflexology schools in the late 1960s (Mackereth & O'Hara 2002).

In practice, the majority of reflexology treatments are provided in the community, either in private clinics or a patient's home. Reflexology, in common with other touch-based interventions, is usually carried out on a one-to-one basis, requiring weekly appointments. Sessions typically involve hands-on treatment lasting 45–50 minutes. The process includes cleaning the feet, applying either talc or small amounts of moisturising cream/quality vegetable oil, and making physical contact by using relaxing manoeuvres. These include holding and stroking the feet, rotating the ankles and toes and stretching various parts of the feet. Integral to the therapy is a map of the feet (see Figures 14.1 and 14.2) which reflexologists use to guide their treatment (Norman 1992). Both feet are usually palpated using thumb and finger pressure, pressing on all areas of the feet and focusing on specific areas of the feet that are tender or sensitive. The session typically ends with 'solar plexus breathing', which uses a specific point and a series of deep breaths. Patients are commonly advised to attend a minimum of six sessions, as benefits are argued to be cumulative (Norman 1992).

Reflexology is viewed as a treatment rather than a set of techniques. It usually encompasses privacy of the interaction, the communication skills of the therapist, and an intention to promote relaxation and improved wellbeing (O'Hara 2002). The semi-recumbent position for the patient is routine and allows for face-to-face contact and conversation. The interaction between therapist and patient includes feedback on the pressure used as well as opportunities for dialogue regarding the patient's health concerns and treatment expectations. There is potential for reflexology, with its series of treatments, to evolve as a supportive event which patients look forward to.

Modern reflexologists do not claim to cure illnesses. They believe that reflexology can help in symptom management (Kunz & Kunz 1993). Ernst and Koder (1997) report that reflexology is rapidly becoming one of the most

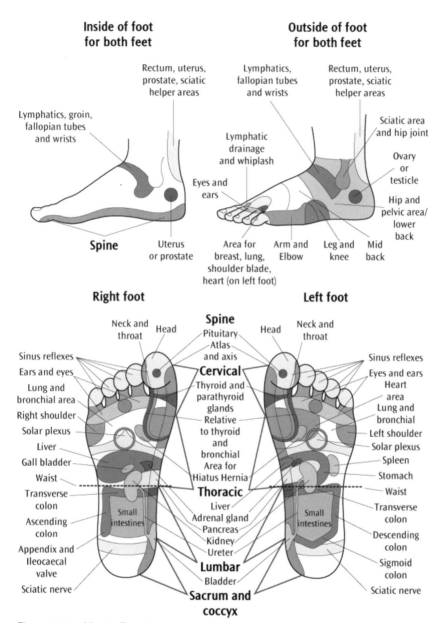

**Inside of foot
for both feet**

Rectum, uterus,
prostate, sciatic
helper areas

Lymphatics, groin,
fallopian tubes
and wrists

Spine

Uterus
or prostate

**Outside of foot
for both feet**

Lymphatics,
fallopian tubes
and wrists

Rectum, uterus,
prostate, sciatic
helper areas

Lymphatic
drainage
and whiplash

Eyes and
ears

Sciatic area
and hip joint

Ovary
or
testicle

Hip and
pelvic area/
lower
back

Area for
breast, lung,
shoulder blade,
heart (on left foot)

Arm and
Elbow

Leg and
knee

Mid
back

Right foot

Neck and
throat

Head

Sinus reflexes

Ears and eyes

Lung and
bronchial area

Right shoulder

Solar plexus

Liver

Gall bladder

Waist

Transverse
colon

Ascending
colon

Appendix and
Ileocaecal
valve

Sciatic nerve

Small
intestines

Spine

Pituitary

Atlas

and axis

Cervical

Thyroid and
parathyroid
glands

Relative
to thyroid
and
bronchial

Area for
Hiatus Hernia

Thoracic

Liver

Adrenal gland

Pancreas

Kidney

Ureter

Lumbar

Bladder

**Sacrum and
coccyx**

Left foot

Head

Neck and
throat

Sinus reflexes

Eyes and ears

Heart
area

Lung and
bronchial

Left shoulder

Solar plexus

Spleen

Stomach

Waist

Transverse
colon

Descending
colon

Sigmoid
colon

Sciatic nerve

Small
intestines

Figure 14.1 Map 1: Foot chart.

popular complementary therapies in the UK, increasingly recommended by
general practitioners (GPs) (White et al 1997), with many nurses and midwives
working towards greater integration within their own practice (Dryden et al
1998, Tiran 1996). Internationally, reflexology is achieving greater integration
in healthcare. In Denmark, for example, reflexology is the most frequently
used complementary therapy funded by the state (Launso et al 1999).

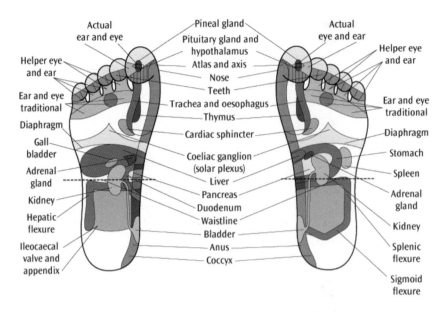

Right foot

Left foot

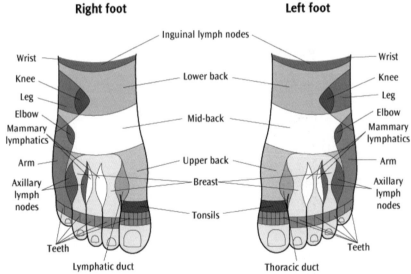

Figure 14.2   Map 2: Reflexology foot chart.

BENEFITS AND CHALLENGES OF REFLEXOLOGY

There are many reasons for the suitability and popularity of reflexology in a cancer care setting. As an intervention involving touch, mostly to the feet, the patient can remain fully dressed, so treatment can be both non-threatening and pleasant to receive. Reflexology can be a useful starting point from which to introduce touch as a therapy. As the therapist is usually face-to-face with the patient, there is also potential for engagement in conversation, providing opportunities to share fears and anxieties and ask for advice; this has been reported in the literature (Gambles 2002). The patient's condition can vary throughout the cancer journey and also from day to day (Hodkinson & Williams 2002). A skilled therapist will need the ability to assess the patient's condition, taking into consideration any cautions and identify potential contraindications. The ability to adapt the techniques and skills to the individual patient is essential to provide a safe and potent treatment. The advantages and challenges of reflexology in cancer care settings are summarised in Box 14.1.

EVIDENCE FOR BENEFIT OF REFLEXOLOGY IN CANCER CARE

The benefits of using reflexology in this type of setting can be wide ranging, as reflexology claims to have effects on the physical body and also in helping to balance the whole person. For example, reflexology can be a way to allow safe release of suppressed emotions, especially with the support of

---

Box 14.1
The advantages and challenges of reflexology

Advantages

- Access is usually through the feet so there is no need for the patient to undress.
- Hands and ears (auricular reflexology) can also be used thus offering a choice of access.
- Patient is usually treated in a semi-recumbent position which facilitates space for conversation.
- Short treatments can be given for specific problems, e.g. nausea, pain, anxiety.
- Patients can be taught to self-treat using their own hands. This may, for example, be helpful prior to receiving chemotherapy or attending a potentially stressful appointment.
- Carers can learn to supplement the therapist's treatment but within limits.

Challenges

- The theoretical basis for reflexology is not fully understood or researched.
- Some reflexologists view the diagnosis of cancer as a contraindication.
- Health professionals may be sceptical of claimed benefits.
- Patients may be sensitive or embarrassed about their feet.
- Hands and ears are often underused by reflexologists.
- The interactive and tactile nature of the therapy may provide a space for sharing of worries and concerns, possibly leading to emotional release.
- Patients with altered sensation may have difficulties providing feedback to the therapist.
- Disease progression may compromise the skin and soft tissues (e.g. lymphoedema, altered sensation, clotting disorders and immunosuppression).

an empathic and skilled therapist (Mackereth 1999). Anecdotal evidence and some small research studies suggest that reflexology can help with many cancer and treatment-related symptoms, such as pain, discomfort, lethargy (see Chapter 3).

Although there is an increasing amount of literature reporting reflexology use in patients while having treatments such as chemotherapy, radiotherapy (Hodkinson 2005, Hodkinson & Williams 2002, Kassab & Stevensen 1996), there is concern among therapists and other healthcare professionals that they may affect the spread of cancer by using reflexology or even working over a reflex area that corresponds to a tumour site. There is no evidence to support that reflexology (or massage) might contribute to the progression of cancer (Hodkinson 2005, MacDonald 1999, McNamara 1993). In continuous professional development workshops for reflexologists, many have expressed worry about the potential detoxification of the body following reflexology treatments, resulting in the decreased effectiveness of cytotoxic drugs. Although some schools teach that reflexology is primarily a stimulating and detoxifying treatment, current literature suggests that it is a treatment that balances the whole body, helping it to achieve its own equilibrium or homeostasis (O'Hara 2002). There has been no published evidence, anecdotal or otherwise, to suggest cytotoxic drugs being rendered less effective following reflexology.

Other fears relate to the potential contamination of the therapist's hands from contact with the by-products of cytotoxic drugs through the sweat glands in the patient's skin. It is important to acknowledge that cytotoxic drugs are metabolised by the liver and rendered less active, subsequently the by-products are excreted in the faeces and urine (Dougherty & Bailey 2001). Unless the practitioner is handling body fluids or the drugs themselves, contamination through the skin is unlikely, especially if the treatment is followed by thorough handwashing procedures. Again there have been no published reports of adverse reaction from reflexology with a patient who is having chemotherapy. Indeed, patients frequently report reduction in the side effects of treatments (e.g. nausea and vomiting) and an increase in relaxation (Hodkinson 2005). Patients also acknowledge the support given by reflexology during difficult and debilitating treatment regimens, and feel that it has been a significant factor in helping them to cope.

Some reflexologists are wary of treating a patient who is having radiotherapy treatment. Radiotherapists support the view that at the end of each radiotherapy treatment there is no residual radioactive material in the patient that could contaminate others. Reflexology can be very supportive to a patient undergoing radiotherapy treatments in terms of helping to manage side effects and from an emotional perspective. It is important to report a study by Grace Smith (2002) investigating the benefits of reflexology for women with breast cancer (n = 150) receiving radiotherapy. There were significant differences for both reflexology and foot massage (given by the same therapist) compared with standard care in some subscales of the mood scale and fatigue checklist.

For reflexology there was a trend for a possible effect on lymphocyte activity worthy of further investigation (Smith 2002).

ABSOLUTE CONTRAINDICATIONS

Skilled and experienced therapists can work in a wide range of situations, adapting their treatments to work safely and potently to suit the individual. There are recognised cautions and conditions of which therapists will need to be aware in order to adapt a particular treatment, e.g. deep vein thrombosis, neuropathy, low platelet count, lymphoedema (Tavares 2003). Absolute contraindications are usually those surrounding consent, for example where a patient is not capable or competent to give consent. Infection risk may also need to be considered if the patient has a severely compromised immune system. If in doubt the therapist must always consult with the patient's medical and nursing team. Consideration also needs to be given to patients with highly resistant infections and radium implants. A therapist would need to refer to hospital policy and to departmental procedure before making contact with the patient and giving a treatment.

Many factors affect the nature of the reflexes of the feet and their condition must be taken into consideration when assessing a patient and planning a treatment. The reflexes of the feet can be affected in many ways. Drugs such as strong analgesics, hypnotics, steroids, tranquillisers and cytotoxic drugs can alter sensation in the feet causing reduced sensitivity, or occasionally with some cytotoxic drugs, hypersensitivity. Chronic illness, emotional and physical pain can also affect sensitivity in reflexes, as can tumours of the central nervous system, neuropathy and other non-cancer-related conditions such as multiple sclerosis and stroke (Tavares 2003).

POSITIONING OF PATIENTS FOR REFLEXOLOGY

As each patient is individual, so is his or her treatment. When working with advanced cancers, it is often necessary for the therapists to consider the comfort of the patient and be willing to be flexible and imaginative in the adaptation of a treatment. Due to the nature of the treatment, reflexology can be given anywhere providing the reflexes are accessible. Patients can be treated in bed (either in a clinical setting or at home), in an armchair or wheelchair, in the garden on a summer day or in a specially designated treatment area. Reflexology does not always necessitate a treatment room, but privacy and a therapeutic environment can facilitate relaxation and communication. A patient with severe weight changes, poor nutrition and poor skin integrity may be at risk from developing pressure sores. Pillows and aids for relieving pressure may be needed to protect vulnerable bony prominences and pressure areas.

When giving a reflexology treatment, patients will need to be in a position best suited to their individual needs. For example, a patient with a sacral pressure sore or a sacral tumour or who is uncomfortable lying on their back, can be treated whilst lying on their front (see Case study 14.1). The feet can also be supported by pillows or a patient could lie on their side, again using pillows to provide support (see Figures 14.3 and 14.4).

Case study 14.1

Tom, aged 33, had a sarcoma of his lumbar spine and sacral area. It had become increasingly more uncomfortable for Tom to have reflexology in the conventional position with him lying semi-supine on a reclining chair. The therapist assisted Tom to lie on his side on the treatment couch. He was supported by a pillow between his legs and another one close to his chest which he was able to hug. He found this position extremely comfortable and subsequently slept throughout most of the treatment.

A breathless patient may be more comfortable when sitting upright or in a high side-lying position (requires an adjustable back rest and support pillows). If available, a bed table can be used with pillows and the patient leaning forward in the orthopnoeic position. Care must be taken not to over-engage a breathless patient in conversation. In many situations the patient is most likely to be treated by the bedside, either in a chair or in bed. Therapists must ensure the patient is comfortable without compromising their own posture (Pyves & Mackereth 2002). When treating a patient in bed, many therapists find it useful to remove the bed end to facilitate easier access to the feet. Due to the close proximity of other patients and visitors, privacy and intrusive background noise can often be an issue. Therapists also have to take

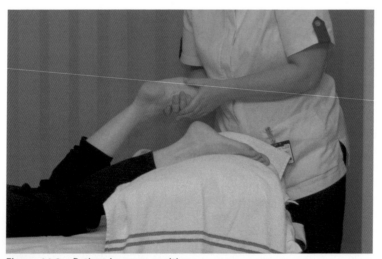

Figure 14.3 Patient in prone position.

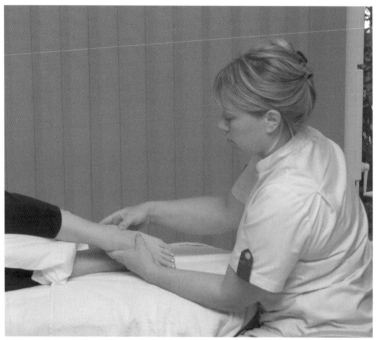

Figure 14.4   Patient in side-lying position.

into account the presence of a urinary catheter, intravenous infusions/devices, anti-embolism stockings, dressings, nasogastric tubes, and oxygen therapy. In cancer settings, it is also not uncommon for patients to be troubled by nausea, vomiting and the need to expectorate. There may also be interruptions when health professionals need to monitor and administer treatments to a patient.

INNOVATIVE TECHNIQUES

In working in cancer care settings a 'no pain, no gain' approach to reflexology has no place. Deep pressure techniques such as Advanced Reflexology Techniques (Porter 1996) or Rwo Shur (Wade 2005) that include deep tissue work using knuckles, constant pressure, the use of implements or 'invigorating' techniques would be inappropriate in a cancer setting. These techniques may present a risk to underlying soft tissue and fragile skin; they could also cause unnecessary distress and pain to the patient. Light gentle touch techniques have been advocated by numerous reflexologists, including Pat Morrell and Chris Stormer (Griffiths 1996). These techniques can involve gentle finger and thumb rolling, rotation, stroking, pulsing and light holding. Gentle reflexology is more commonly used in palliative and cancer care settings. Not only is it safer in terms of reducing trauma to skin and soft tissue, but it can be useful in managing physical symptoms. Light touch can be profound in its effects on psychological wellbeing through promoting relaxation and pain relief. Examples of innovative uses of reflexology are given in Table 14.1.

Table 14.1
Innovative reflexology techniques for patients with cancer

Techniques	Description	Aims/indications	Therapist's activity	Patient/carer involvement
Precision Reflexology Developed by Jan Williamson and Prue Miskin	Gentle linking of specific reflexology points Techniques can involve stillness and focus. Specific areas of the body such as the endocrine system and Chakras of body are treated. Links can also involve bony structures and organs of the body	Relaxation and stress reduction Aim is to restore balance, harmony and energy flow. Can be used in patients who are fatigued	'Linking' or holding two or more reflex points, i.e. lung and spine area The therapist tunes in the energy felt between the links and holds and listens to the energy response. Can be incorporated with other reflexology approaches	Patients are encouraged to rest, but can give feedback Can be used as a self-help technique on the hands by patients. Carers can be taught simple 'links', under the supervision of a suitably qualified therapist
AirReflexology© Developed by Edwina Hodkinson and Barbara Cook	Involves combining reflexology theory and map to provide 'off the skin' or energy field reflexology	Avoids skin contact/ physical pressure. May be useful when the feet are sensitive to touch, oedema and/or bruising or skin damage, methicillin resistant *Staphylococcus aureus* (MRSA) infection. Patient needs to be comfortable and open to the concept of energy medicine	Therapist needs to be calm, receptive and centred Hands are placed 2–4 cm above the skin Movements over the feet and hands can be flowing, stationary (holding) and/or multidirectional Movements can involve circling, pulling away, tapping, fanning. Assessment and treatment take place simultaneously and intuitively	Patient can rest or give feedback Visualisation and gentle breathing techniques can be offered Intention is to help without imposing the therapist's own beliefs or judgements. Patients and/or formal and informal carers can be taught simple techniques
HypnoReflexology© Developed by Peter Mackereth and Paula Maycock	Deep relaxation techniques using breath work, pressure point work combined with	To provide the patients with empowering techniques and anchors to manage anxieties	The work can be planned to occur outside or within a stressful or phobic situation (e.g. needle phobia or anticipatory nausea and vomiting)	Patients and carers can be taught self-help techniques, with tapes and instruction sheets provided

	controlled use of the voice, safe space, and anchoring techniques to help with distressing anxieties, phobias and symptoms (e.g. pain, nausea)	and phobias in the context of a reflexology session	Reflexology techniques are incorporated to deepen relaxation and assist with symptom management	
Creative Relaxation Reflexology (CRR) Barbara Cook	Combines gentle reflexology with creative imagery and visualisation	Promotes relaxation, particularly with patients who are anxious, fearful or find it hard to let go of tension. The technique also facilitates connection with the whole body, and so enhances the treatment process. Relaxation music can be used to support the work	The therapist invites creation of a relaxing place to visit. Using the reflexology map gentle touch techniques are used to encourage the patient to bring attention to and relax the body area being worked	The patient can take an active part in creating the journey and place Alternatively the therapist can offer a guided imagery using a choice of scripted scenes (i.e. beach or garden). Patient can choose their own music
Four-Hands Holding Reflexology (Mackereth et al 2000)	Involves two qualified therapists working in synergy with a patient	Promotes relaxation, provides nurturing environment. Intensifies use of touch so can reduce treatment time. Can be used as teaching technique, especially when working with new therapists or carers	Therapists can either work both feet together or treat opposite polarities of the body, such as feet and hands or feet and the head. It is important that one person takes the lead, their role being to introduce the approach and to lead the treatment for the other therapist to follow, mirror or anchor (e.g. support/hold the head)	Patient can remain passive, giving feedback Carers can be paired with the therapist It is important to ensure that both carer and patients are comfortable with this technique*

*See guidance in Chapter 7.

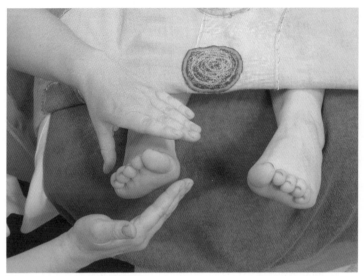

Figure 14.5   AirReflexology©.

Consideration and support needs to be given to patients who undergo cathartic release during therapy, allowing them time and permission to safely express release of emotions in a nurturing environment. Light touch can also incorporate 'AirReflexology©', which utilises the reflexology map (see Figures 14.1 and 14.2) to provide 'off the skin' or energy field reflexology (see Figure 14.5). These techniques can be useful with patients who have very painful or sensitive reflexes, neuropathy, petechial haemorrhage, lymphoedema or skin problems (see Case study 14.2).

Case study 14.2

Val, aged 55, was receiving chemotherapy for leukaemia. She requested reflexology because she was feeling very low and anxious. She was thrombocytopenic and staff expressed concern with treatment due to the risk of bruising. Following discussion it was agreed to provide AirReflexology© over the feet. Val was delighted to be allowed some form of treatment. The therapist worked 'off the skin' using stroking and circular movements focusing on imbalanced reflexes using small circular movements and linking techniques. Val relaxed immediately and said she felt as though her skin was being touched gently by a soothing breeze. She reported sleeping serenely and later awaking refreshed.

Precision Reflexology is another useful approach advocated by Jan Williamson and Prue Miskin (Williamson 1999) that involves gentle 'linking' of specific reflexology points (see Figure 14.6). As it aims to restore energy and promotes deep relaxation it is ideal for patients who are fatigued and anxious (see Case study 14.3).

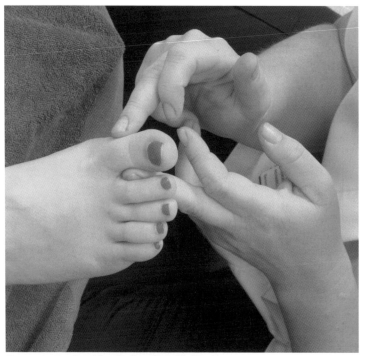

Figure 14.6   Precision Reflexology 'linking'.

Case study 14.3

Karen, aged 45, had advanced ovarian cancer with extensive pelvic metastasis and severe bilateral lymphoedema in her legs. Karen felt tired and anxious and wanted to have work done on her feet, as they felt heavy and cold. Adaptation to the reflexology included a combination of Precision Reflexology and AirReflexology©. Karen relaxed immediately and reported tingling and lightness in her legs. She felt very peaceful and commented to her husband afterwards how wonderful she felt.

WORKING WITH CARERS

A diagnosis of cancer and a poor prognosis can be very distressing, not only for the patient, but also for those involved in supporting and caring for them. It can reduce their energy levels and increase anxiety (Aranda & Hayman-White 2001). Receiving a reflexology treatment can help carers to take time out and to focus on their own needs. It can provide an opportunity for carers to talk about their feelings, to help them to manage their own anxiety and stress and to deal with issues that they feel unable to talk about to their loved ones (Hodkinson & Williams 2002). Many carers have a range of health concerns of their own, which may have been precipitated or exacerbated by the caring burden. Reflexology can help in coping with and managing health problems and provides a safe environment in which to receive support.

USING 'FOUR-HANDS HOLDING' WITH CARERS

Some carers may find help in the relief of their own stress and anxiety through being involved in the patient's reflexology treatment. Carers can feel that they are making a contribution if they are taught a simple and safe complementary therapy treatment which can be given to the patient or are involved in a treatment provided by the therapist (see Chapter 7).

Four-Hands Holding is where two therapists or a therapist and carer work with an individual simultaneously (see Figure 14.7 and Table 14.1). An example of Four-Hands Holding could involve a carer gently massaging the patient's hands (having learnt a simple routine), while the therapist works the patient's feet. However, it is important for the therapist to be aware that the carer may be uncomfortable with this type of touch, and there should be no pressure on the carer to participate. It is important to ask for feedback from the carer after the treatment. As this may be a new experience, responses can range from feeling that they have contributed to care and comfort, to being moved, and even a little tearful from the experience.

One of the authors of this chapter, Barbara Cook (see Table 14.1), has developed an approach that combines gentle reflexology with guided visualisations, which includes using the reflexology map to encourage relaxation in the various parts of the body. Another approach that combines reflexology and deep relaxation techniques has been termed 'HypnoReflexology©' (see Table 14.1). This intervention has been developed in an acute cancer setting and requires further training and ongoing supervision. It is particularly useful

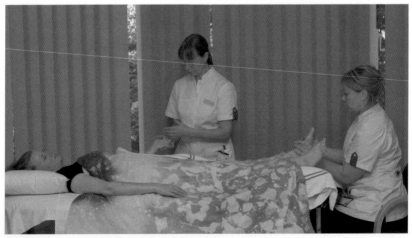

Figure 14.7   Four-Hands Holding Reflexology technique.

for a patient receiving chemotherapy, who might be experiencing distressing responses to treatments, such as anticipatory nausea and vomiting and needle phobia (see Case study 14.4).

Case study 14.4

Derek, aged 45, had bowel cancer and was attending weekly for chemotherapy. It was his third treatment and he was unable to enter the chemo-suite because of overwhelming anxiety and nausea. He was hyperventilating and clutching a vomit bowl. Derek was offered the option of seeing a reflexologist. Eager to try anything he agreed. The therapist worked reflexology areas for stress and digestion while guiding Derek to visualise and describe a safe place. He chose a beach with palm trees, golden sands and an aqua blue sea. Derek could even describe feeling a light breeze and the warm sun on his skin. He worked with his symptoms (nausea) by using a 'volume control'. Once the lowest score was achieved Derek anchored the safe place and calm state by placing the right hand on his forearm. Derek could then use this to anchor the experience for future use. Within 10 minutes he was calmer, the vomit bowl was on the floor and the chemo nurse had inserted an intravenous (IV) line on first attempt.

At home Derek practised the techniques (including reflexology self-help points on the hands), using a relaxation tape and with the support of his partner. The therapist made a point of being available for Derek's next visit to the chemo-suite and noted that he was calmer and less nauseated, and he only needed a short treatment to facilitate the insertion of the IV line.

Box 14.2
Recommendations for reflexology and cancer care

- A diagnosis of cancer is not a contraindication for reflexology, but care must be taken with adapting classical techniques to ensure comfort and safety.
- Patients with lymphoedema require careful assessment by a lymphoedema specialist before considering any reflexology interventions.
- AirReflexology© and linking techniques may be ideal adaptations with compromised skin as they avoid direct tissue pressure.
- Short and gentle treatments using light touch will help avoid tiredness in fatigued patients.
- Carers and patients can be taught simple interventions, which can be used with the hands.
- If the condition of the feet (e.g. altered sensation, localised infection, amputation, lymphoedema of the feet) precludes reflexology the hands or ears could be considered as an alternative.

SUMMARY

The chapter explored approaches to reflexology that are both innovative and mindful of the patient's symptoms and safety. Recommendations for working in cancer care settings are detailed in Box 14.2. It is important to recognise that this work requires further training, support and supervision to skilfully adapt the treatment.

REFERENCES

Aranda SK, Hayman-White K 2001 Home caregivers of the person with advanced cancer. An Australian perspective. Cancer Nursing 24(4):300–307

Dougherty L, Bailey C 2001 Chemotherapy. In: Corner J, Bailey C (eds) Cancer nursing: care in context. Blackwell Science, Oxford

Dryden S, Holden S, Mackereth P 1998 'Just the ticket'; integrating massage and reflexology in practice (Part 1). Complementary Therapies in Nursing and Midwifery 4(6):154–159

Ernst E, Koder K 1997 Reflexology: an overview. European Journal of General Practice 3:52–57

Gambles M, Crooke M, Wilkinson S 2002 Evaluation of a hospice based reflexology service: a qualitative audit of patient perceptions. European Journal of Oncology Nursing 6(1):37–44

Graham L, Goldstone L, Ejindu A et al 1998 Penetration of complementary therapies into NHS trust and private hospital practice. Complementary Therapies in Nursing and Midwifery 4(6):160–165

Griffiths P 1996 Reflexology. In: Rankin-Box D (ed) The nurse's handbook of complementary therapies. Churchill Livingstone, London

Hodkinson E 2005 Reflexology for people with cancer. Reflexions, June edn, pp. 2–5

Hodkinson E, Williams J 2002 Enhancing quality of life for people in palliative care settings. In: Mackereth P, Tiran D (eds) Clinical reflexology: a guide for health professionals. Churchill Livingstone, Edinburgh

Kassab S, Stevensen C 1996 Common misunderstandings about complementary therapies for people with cancer. Complementary Therapies in Nursing and Midwifery 2(3):62–65

Kohn M 1999 Complementary Therapies in Cancer Care. Macmillan Cancer Relief, London

Kunz K, Kunz B 1993 The complete guide to foot reflexology (revised). Kunz & Kunz, Albuquerque, TX

Launso L, Brendstrup E, Arnberg S 1999 An exploratory study of reflexological treatment for headache. Alternative Therapies 5(3):57–65

MacDonald G 1999 Medicine hands, massage therapy for people with cancer. Findhorne Press, Tallahassee, FL

Mackereth PA 1999 An introduction to catharsis and the healing crisis in reflexology. Complementary Therapies in Nursing and Midwifery 5(3):67–74

Mackereth P, O'Hara C 2002 Preparatory and continuing education. In: Mackereth P, Tiran D (eds) Clinical reflexology: a guide for health professionals. Churchill Livingstone, Edinburgh

Mackereth P, Campbell G, Norman M et al 2000 Introducing '4-Hands Holding': many hands make profound work. Cahoots 72:36–38

McNamara P 1993 Massage for people with cancer. Wandsworth Cancer Support Centre, London

Norman L 1992 The reflexology handbook – a complete guide. Piatkus, London

O'Hara C 2002 Challenging the 'rules' of reflexology. In: Mackereth P, Tiran D (eds) Clinical reflexology: a guide for health professionals. Churchill Livingstone, Edinburgh

Porter AJ 2002 The ART Manual. AJ Porter Publishing, London

Pyves G, Mackereth P 2002 Practising safely and effectively: introducing the 'No Hands' approach, a paradigm shift in the theory and practice of reflexology. In: Mackereth P, Tiran D (eds) Clinical reflexology: a guide for health professionals. Churchill Livingstone, Edinburgh

Smith G 2002 A randomised controlled clinical trial of reflexology in breast cancer patients, to reduce fatigue resulting from radiotherapy to the breast and chest wall. PhD thesis, University of Liverpool, Liverpool

Tavares M 2003 The National Guidelines for the Use of Complementary Therapies in Supportive and Palliative Care. The Prince's Foundation for Integrated Health, National Council for Hospice and Specialist Palliative Care Services, London

Tiran D 1996 The use of complementary therapies in midwifery practice: a focus on reflexology. Complementary Therapies in Nursing and Midwifery 2(2): 32–37

Wade N 2005 Taiwanese reflexology – Father Josef Method also known as Rwo Shur. Reflexions, p. 11

White AR, Resch K-L, Ernst E 1997 Complementary medicine: use and attitudes by GPs. Family Practitioner 14:302–306

Williamson J 1999 A guide to precision reflexology. Mark Allen Publishing, Bath

FURTHER READING

Mackereth PA, Tiran D (eds) Clinical reflexology: a guide for health professionals. Churchill Livingstone, Edinburgh

Pyves G 2005 In celebration of feet. Shi'Zen Publications, Hebden Bridge, Yorkshire, UK

USEFUL ADDRESSES

Edwina Hodkinson
Deputy Clinical Lead for Complementary Therapies
Christie Hospital NHS Trust
c/o The Rehabilitation Unit
Wilmslow Road
Manchester M20 4BX
UK

Barbara Cook
Beechwood Cancer Care Centre
Chelford Grove, Adswood
Stockport SK3 8LS
UK

Adapting chair massage for carers, staff and patients

15

Gwynneth Campbell, Peter A Mackereth and Paola Sylt

Abstract

Chair massage is becoming increasingly popular in the workplace and other social settings. This chapter explores and describes a project set up to provide the intervention in cancer care to patients, carers and staff. More specifically the authors report on findings from service audit and evaluation of a carers' service.

KEYWORDS

chair massage, training, evaluation, carers, patients, staff

INTRODUCTION

There is growing evidence of the benefits of chair massage among healthcare staff in terms of wellbeing and improving alertness, and alleviating tiredness and fatigue. Massage is traditionally given in the supine position in therapy rooms, with hourly appointments. The ergonomically designed massage chair provides an opportunity for short, seated, clothed treatments. Evidence is presented in this chapter for its efficacy and need for adaptation for patients with cancer and their visiting relatives. First is a brief history of chair massage, followed by a description of specialised training and service evaluation. Aside from presentation of data, case studies and recommendation for best practice are also given.

HISTORY OF CHAIR MASSAGE

The therapeutic use of massage has been recognised for thousands of years and practised worldwide in a variety of cultures and forms, including in the seated position. In healthcare settings physiotherapists, and occasionally nurses, have massaged a sitting patient's neck and shoulders by asking him or

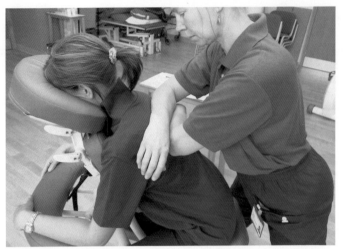

Figure 15.1   Massage chair supporting the whole body.

her to lean forward over a bed-table piled with pillows (Holey & Cook 2003). David Palmer, an experienced massage instructor, developed a form of seated massage in the 1980s using elements of acupressure and meridian theory that could be done anywhere, using an ergonomically designed and portable padded foldable chair (Palmer 1998). The chair supports the whole body (Figure 15.1), and conveniently allows the client to relax and receive a fully clothed massage without the need for oil, bringing the advantages of massage to many people, often for the first time.

There has since been a phenomenal rise of 'on-site' massage in workplaces, airports and healthcare settings. More recently muscle-based techniques have been advocated by chair massage instructors incorporating an innovative approach to prevent injury to practitioners and adapted to the individual client (Greene 1995, Mackereth & Campbell 2002, Pyves & Woodhouse 2003). The adapted chair massage described in this chapter contains elements of both approaches, as well as techniques from other modalities, adapted specifically for use in cancer care settings.

LITERATURE REVIEW

Studies have focused on benefits for workers with limited break time to receive chair massage. Researchers have reported that 15-minute sessions can reduce stress and enhance the electroencephalogram pattern of alertness. A group of workers (n = 26) receiving chair massage twice a week for 5 weeks, studied by Field et al (1996), had more reduced anxiety levels, lowered cortisol readings, improved alertness and higher scores in computational tasks after treatment than the control group (n = 24). An important finding by Cady & Jones (1997) was the significant lowering of both systolic and diastolic blood pressure of employees following a 15-minute on-site massage, but there was no control group in this study. Another relevant study was conducted by Field et al (1997) in which hospital workers were given 10-minute chair massage treatments, afterwards reporting decreases in anxiety, depression and fatigue as well as increases in vigour. Katz et al (1999) conducted a small pilot study evaluating eight sessions of chair massage also given to hospital staff. Relaxation and Profile of Mood States scores were better after the treatment, along with reduction in tension and pain intensity. In a larger study by Hodge et al (2002), involving healthcare workers, subjects were randomised into two groups, one group (n = 50) received 20 minutes of chair massage and the other, the control group (n = 50), rested for an equal time period. Subjects who received chair massage showed decreases in blood pressure, anxiety and sleep disturbances, and improvements in wellbeing and emotional control.

Carers, like staff, often have limited time to receive massage, and may be reluctant to spend time away from loved ones. An evaluation of a service project providing massage to carers in the USA showed that when carers (n = 13) were given an average of six massages, 85% reported emotional and physical stress level reduction, 77% reported physical pain reduction and 54% reported better patterns of sleep (MacDonald 1998). In the UK a massage service for relatives of patients receiving palliative care has been well evaluated by participants in focus groups (Penson 1998). At present there is a paucity of published work evaluating chair massage for patients in supportive and palliative care settings, although there are anecdotal reports of its use (Gray & Mackereth 2003, Holey & Cook 2003).

TRAINING

A specialised chair massage course has been designed specifically for qualified massage therapists who wish to expand their skills in hospice and cancer care (Gray & Mackereth 2003). The comprehensive training includes ways of adapting chair massage for people who are ill, distressed or overburdened by care giving, and to promote safe and effective chair massage practice in supportive and palliative care settings. The programme contains thorough elements on assessment and contracting for chair massage, contraindications and careful adaptations, safety implications and effective use of the chair, as well as a review of research evidence. The practical content looks to safeguard both receiver and therapist, including guidance on posture and safe working (Pyves & Mackereth 2002). For further details see the section Useful address at the end of the chapter.

CHAIR MASSAGE FOR CARERS, PATIENTS AND STAFF

Chair massage can be a way to receive massage safely when privacy is not available and removal of clothing impractical. The portability of the chairs enables therapists to deliver the treatment to the carers wherever they are in the hospital (at the bedside, in dayrooms, drop-in relaxation sessions or even in the gardens). Researchers reviewed a complete year of service provision for carers at Christie Hospital, Manchester, UK and conducted a more formal evaluation through interviews and questionnaires designed to obtain quantitative and qualitative readings and reactions from carers. This is looked at in more detail later in the chapter. It was found that, as the chair massage service for relatives developed, patients themselves began to ask for this treatment. Care needs to be taken in assessing suitability of the chair for patients who have mobility problems, fatigue, severe weight loss and additional problems of equipment, such as intravenous lines and catheters. Initial experience of using the chair with over 50 patients suggests benefits similar to those appreciated by carers (see Box 15.1).

Box 15.1
Reported benefits of chair massage

- Relaxation
- Time for attention and support
- Supported posture
- Assist with pain and muscular stiffness
- Reduced anxiety
- Improvement in mood
- Revitalise and refresh

Mackereth & Campbell (2002).

Healthcare service concerns have been raised about challenging working conditions, high stress levels and problems with sickness and retention for staff and volunteers (Barrett & Yates 2002). Wellbeing days for hospital staff to experience taster sessions of various therapies can be popular (see Figure 15.2).

Although the primary goal of providing a chair massage service for employees and volunteers can help their wellbeing, it can also be a way of promoting the therapeutic use of massage. Once they have experienced it for themselves, healthcare staff will be more aware of the potential of massage services and the benefits, and more likely to refer colleagues, patients and carers for massage themselves. A recent evaluation of complementary therapy services for staff has shown chair massage to be the most popular therapy taken up by staff, and that neck and back pain along with general stress were the most common reasons for self-referral (Mackereth et al 2005).

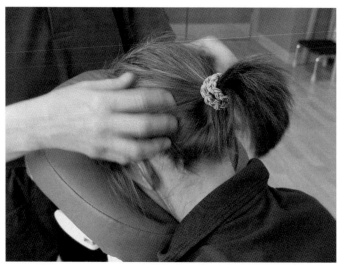

Figure 15.2   A member of staff receiving a taster session of chair massage with head supported on head rest.

APPLICATION TO PRACTICE BASED ON THE CARERS' PROJECT AT CHRISTIE HOSPITAL

This section discusses practice issues in providing treatments for carers. Case studies illustrate individual benefits and experience of the service. Issues related to indications, contraindications and adaptation are examined.

Carers

A process and eventual diagnosis of cancer or any life-threatening or life-limiting disease is not only extremely stressful for patients but also for their families, friends and work colleagues (Faulkner & Maguire 1994, Mackereth & Campbell 2002). All people close to the patient are embarking on the journey as companions, witnessing many investigations, waiting for a diagnosis and seeing at first hand the effects of the disease and the challenges of treatment. Carers have to consider the future, the hope for a cure and also the possibility of losing someone close to them. The journey with cancer and other diseases can involve periods of relapses and remissions, requiring readjustment and revision of hopes and fears. There are practical concerns too, including loss of income because of time away from work or even having to stop work altogether. For carers there is the hospital or hospice bedside vigil, sleeping fitfully on foldaway beds or chairs. Carers literally place their own lives on hold. Attending to everyday personal needs, such as washing hair or having a proper meal, can take irreplaceable time away from being with someone who is very ill and dear to them. Case study 15.1 is an example of such a situation with a carer who was referred for massage by the nursing staff.

Case study 15.1

A patient's partner had been sleeping with considerable discomfort in a chair beside the patient's bed for 2 weeks. He was afraid to leave his partner in case the patient's condition deteriorated. The referral for chair massage was made by one of the ward staff. The carer reported feeling tense and exhausted prior to the massage. His response on a feel-good 'scale' following the 15-minute treatment went from 0 to 10. He reported relaxing completely during the treatment and muscle tension easing. After resting for a few moments he returned to his vigil noticeably refreshed. The next day a member of the nursing team stopped to thank the practitioner, and to report that the patient had died peacefully with the carer awake and calmly present at the bedside.

Much attention has been given to the importance of communicating with carers and providing counselling and pastoral care (Faulkner & Maguire 1994, Robbins 1989) and more recently hospices and cancer care settings have begun to provide complementary therapy for carers, acknowledging they too can benefit from physical interventions. There is increasing recognition of the importance of carers' self-care, and Daniels (2003) suggests that to sustain the carer role it depends on a person's ability to seek out and request the kind of support they need. Chair massage provides another option available within a cancer care setting. As well as healthcare staff initiating referrals, therapists themselves might identify a need and offer chair massage to relatives (see Case study 15.2).

Case study 15.2

Mrs Rose had been maintaining a vigil at her partner's bedside. The therapist first provided a gentle foot massage for Mr Rose and then offered chair massage. She agreed provided she could have the treatment by his bedside. Mrs Rose reported being very anxious and not having slept for the last 2 days. After the treatment she looked much less tense but began to cry. She said the massage had touched her and could no longer hold back the tears.

The visibility of clothed chair massage on an open ward can enable other patients and carers to see it in action, prompting interest in asking for the intervention themselves (see Case study 15.3).

Case study 15.3

In a four-bedded bay a chair massage treatment was being provided to the partner of Mark, a young man with acute spinal cord compression. When his parents arrived to visit him, they appeared anxious and shocked on seeing the deterioration in his condition. On the recommendation of the partner Jane, both received chair massage. After the treatments they appeared calmer and more settled. The patient thanked the two therapists for the attention given to his family. Soon after another patient in the bay requested a treatment for his wife.

Practical considerations and contraindications

Some preparatory considerations before offering chair massage are given in Box 15.2, which contains a series of questions developed from working in clinical settings and gives guidance relating to any form of touch work. It is not prescriptive or an exhaustive list.

Box 15.2
Preparatory considerations

For practitioners to consider about themselves
- Do I have the necessary managerial support and supervision to work with this person?
- Is the space and time available conducive to chair massage?
- Am I calm and centred enough to be present for this person?
- Am I comfortable about asking the recipient for feedback or stopping to clarify the work at any time?

For practitioners to consider about the receivers
- Do they really want to be touched?
- Are they competent, able and willing to consent to the treatment?
- Do they understand my level of skill and the boundaries to this work?
- Are there any impediments to using the massage chair with them?
- Have they reviewed the checklist for contraindications?
- Have arrangements been made to follow-up this session or provide a means of support if needed?

It is important to ensure that referrals comply with existing policy on massage. Then after greeting the carer, the therapist should explain what is being offered, and ask if they would like chair massage. They will need to check contraindications to massage, and assess whether the carer can sit comfortably in the chair for the 15 minutes, before agreeing on content and style of massage. Examples of contraindications are given in Box 15.3.

> **Box 15.3**
> **Examples of contraindications**
>
> - Unable to mount chair
> - Unable to consent, for example confused and disoriented, imbued alcohol, has taken sedatives, strong narcotics or non-prescribed substances
> - Recent surgery or injury
> - Raised temperature or feeling unwell
> - Unstable blood pressure or heart problems
> - Extreme breathlessness
> - Extreme or unexplained pain

Concerns and adaptations

Safety issues in setting up the chair include making adjustments to the height and angle of the seat, headrest and arm rest prior to treatment, ensuring all levers are fixed and pointing away from centre of the chair so they do not harm the carer's body or clothing. Final adjustments to the positioning of the headrest can be made when the carer is seated on the chair. It is important for the recipient to remain comfortable throughout the treatment, and the therapist should tell the recipient to indicate if he or she feels uncomfortable at any time or wants the session to end prematurely.

Ongoing evaluation is crucial and is about the therapist noticing responses to the work, for example relating to depth of breathing or changes in client's muscle tone or skin temperature. Therapists should be considering if they themselves are feeling relaxed and comfortable, and it is very important for therapists to take care of their own bodies while working (Pyves & Mackereth 2002). Figures 15.3 and 15.4 show ways of using the massage chair in a gentle relaxing way, without causing too much strain on the therapist.

Although the massage chair is adaptable, sometimes further considerations are needed. For people using a wheelchair, or those unable to kneel comfortably on the full chair, the half chair is ideal. It consists of a headrest on an adjustable support that rests on a firm surface, like a table or massage couch. Figures 15.5 and 15.6 show the half chair in practice.

Following treatment, recipients of chair massage need time to recover. Offering water and gathering verbal and non-verbal feedback is recommended. Sessions should be evaluated with the carer and confidential documentation maintained. Washing hands, and cleaning the chair, naturally follow.

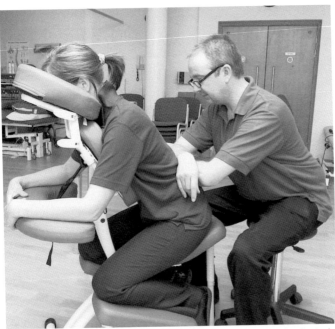

Figure 15.3 Sitting on stool behind the receiver to save back strain while working on lower back.

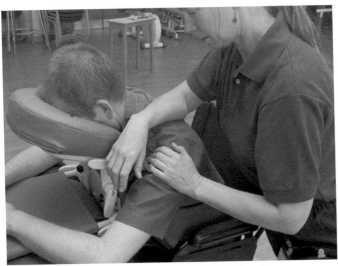

Figure 15.4 Using forearms to save overuse of hands.

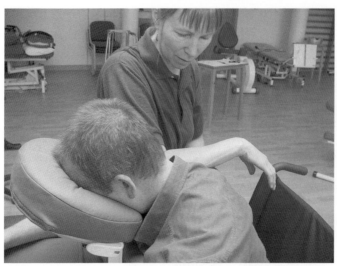

Figure 15.5   Using the half chair, working from side.

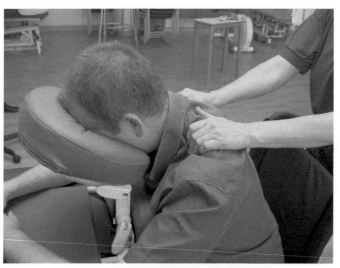

Figure 15.6   Using the half chair, working from behind.

EVALUATION OF THE CARERS' PROJECT

An important goal for supportive and palliative care services to fulfil the recommendations of The Cancer Plan (Department of Health 2000) is to evaluate
complementary therapies for patients and also for carers. Audits being conducted at Christie Hospital aim to evaluate the current provision of the carers'
service.

Permission had been obtained to use Tiffany Field's 'Feeling Good Thermometer', a visual analogue scale to evaluate wellbeing before and after therapeutic interventions (Field 2000). This is a way of recording the subjective feel-good factor on a scale of 0–10 (0 being 'not feeling good at all' and 10 being the 'best I've ever felt'). Preliminary findings indicated that informal carers were reporting reduction in anxiety, pain and muscular stiffness, increase in relaxation, time for attention and support, improvement in mood and feeling revitalised and refreshed (Mackereth & Campbell 2003). Hence, a formal study was conducted during 2004 to evaluate the effects of the massage service and obtain a measure of:

- Relief from physical ailments, such as muscular stiffness and pain, headaches, fatigue and lack of sleep.
- Relief from psychological stresses, such as anxiety, depression, sorrow, helplessness and worry.

In addition, the evaluation looked at 'next day' response patterns, to see if the benefits continued to exert effects beyond the immediate possible halo effects of the treatment, in particular any changes in sleep, fatigue, worry and anxiety. Furthermore, participants in this study had 24 hours to think about whether they would wish to receive the massage again and to offer comments and critique regarding the service. This was in line with recommendations from the National Institute for Clinical Excellence (NICE 2003), which suggested that cancer services be evaluated to identify models of service that are acceptable and helpful to carers.

The published project comprised two stages (Mackereth et al 2005). The first involved a review of the records of 182 informal carers who had received treatments of chair massage during the previous 12 months. A significant increase in general wellbeing was noted ($p < 0.001$), with 97% of carers having reported an improvement. Stage 2 randomly recruited 34 relatives and close friends of inpatients at the hospital, who were receiving the massage on a voluntary basis during the course of a week. A brief interview was conducted after the massage and a short questionnaire was given to each participant to self-complete the following day. As previously found, results revealed significant improvements in both physical ($p < 0.001$) and psychological ($p < 0.001$) wellbeing, with 97% of carers registering physical improvements, e.g. increased muscular mobility and energy levels with reduction in pain and tension, and 70% an improvement in their emotional state, e.g. relaxation, calm and reduced feelings of anxiety and worry. In addition, a good level of both physical ($p < 0.001$) and psychological ($p < 0.002$) improvements appeared to have been retained a day after the massage.

The study also found that a large number of participants seemed to have improved their sleep pattern on the night after the massage and reduced levels of worry were registered. As good sleep represents a valuable source of energy, improved sleep patterns would support the reported retained effects of the massage. During the study it was observed that the massage had been generally valued and enjoyed, and this could be seen by the participants regretting the end of the session and wishing to repeat the experience, possibly on a daily basis. It was also noted that, through receiving the massage the carers became more aware of any postural problems, caused by tension or long hours by the bedside. During interviews carers frequently reported that they were suffering from physical discomfort or pain to the upper body, often aggravated by the stressful role of being a carer. The majority of carers seemed to 'house' feelings of emotional tension and burden on head, neck and shoulders. As these areas were the main focus of the massage treatment, the intervention seemed to demonstrate having provided great relief to physical areas of concern, as well as having provided relaxation and emotional release.

This project revealed that female carers and parents of patients had received, and retained to the following day, the highest level of benefit from the treatment. This is particularly significant, as they appeared to be the most vulnerable and needy groups of carers by displaying the lowest pre-massage levels of both physical and psychological wellbeing. These findings would enhance the positive evaluation of the massage service and suggest that this type of treatment could be well suited to provide support to these groups of carers, perhaps with a more sustained method of delivery.

The massage offered an action that communicates love, support and acceptance. It appeared to be giving the carers the opportunity to feel valued and the confidence to recognise and voice their own needs, an indication that carers need to be asked about their issues, which would otherwise remain unrecognised. By being encouraged to look after their own health and to try to meet their own needs, carers would hopefully gain wellbeing and would feel more able to cope with the caring role, which would be clearly beneficial to themselves and to the person they are supporting.

SUMMARY

This chapter has shown how chair massage has developed and can be a valuable tool for a complementary therapy service in a hospital setting. The training and development of a service for patients, staff and carers has been discussed. Practical considerations have been addressed, and the importance of evaluating projects. Case studies and results from the evaluation of the chair project for carers at Christie Hospital indicate the extent of the benefits to the carers both physically and emotionally.

REFERENCES

Barrett L, Yates P 2002 Oncology haematology nurses: a study of job satisfaction, burnout and intention to leave the speciality. Australian Health Review 25(3):109–121

Cady SH, Jones GE 1997 Massage therapy as a workplace intervention for reduction of stress. Perceptual & Motor Skills 84(1):157–158

Daniels R 2003 The carer's guide in cancer lifeline kit. Health Creation, Bristol

Department of Health 2000 The NHS cancer plan: a plan for investment. A plan for reform. The Stationery Office, London

Faulkner A, Maguire P 1994 Talking to cancer patients and their relatives. Oxford University Press, Oxford

Field T 2000 Touch therapy. Churchill Livingstone, London

Field T, Ironson G, Scafidid F et al 1996 Massage therapy reduces anxiety and enhances EEG pattern of alertness and maths computations. International Journal of Neurosciences 86(3–4):197–205

Field T, Quintino O, Henteleff Wells-Keife L et al 1997 Job stress reduction therapies. Alternative Therapies 3(4):54–56

Gray D, Mackereth P 2003 Complementary therapies at Christie Hospital. Body & Soul, Spring edn, pp. 15–16

Greene L 1995 Save your hands. Gilded Age Press, Florida

Hodge M, Robinson C, Boehmer J 2002 Employee outcomes following work-site acupressure and massage. Massage Therapy Journal 39(3):48–64

Holey E, Cook E 2003 Evidence-based therapeutic massage: a practical guide for therapists, 2nd edn. Churchill Livingstone, London

Katz J, Wowk A, Culp D et al 1999 Pain and tension are reduced among hospital nurses after on-site massage treatments: a pilot study. Journal of Perianesthesia Nursing 14(3):128–133

MacDonald G 1998 Massage as a respite intervention for primary caregivers. American Journal of Hospice and Palliative Care 15:43–47

Mackereth P, Campbell G 2002 Chair massage: attention and touch in 15 minutes. Palliative and Cancer Matters, issue 25, pp. 2, 6

Mackereth P, Campbell G 2003 Research and chair massage In: Pyves G, Woodhouse D (eds) NOHANDS chair massage. Shizen Publications, Halifax

Mackereth P, Sylt P, Weiberg A et al 2005 Chair massage for carers in an acute cancer hospital. European Journal of Oncology Nursing 9:167–179

NICE 2003 Guidance on cancer services: improving supportive and palliative care for adults with cancer – second consultation draft. NICE, London

Palmer D 1998 Brief history of chair massage. Positive Health, June edn, 32

Penson J 1998 Complementary therapies: making a difference in palliative care. Complementary Therapies in Nursing and Midwifery 4(3):77–81

Pyves G, Mackereth PA 2002 Practising safety and effectively: introducing the 'No Hands' approach, a paradigm shift in the theory and practice of reflexology. In: Mackereth P, Tiran D (eds) Clinical reflexology: a guide for health professionals. Churchill Livingstone, Edinburgh

Pyves G, Woodhouse D (eds) 2003 NOHANDS chair massage. Shizen Publications, Halifax

Robbins J (ed) 1989 Caring for the dying patient and the family. Harper & Row, London

FURTHER READING

Department of Health 2002 Caring about carers: a national strategy for carers. Department of Health, London

Harding R, Higginson IJ 2003 What is the best way to help caregivers in cancer and palliative care? A systematic literature review of interventions and their effectiveness. Palliative Medicine 17(1):63–74

Pyves G 2000 The principles and practice of 'no hands' massage – zero strain bodywork. Shi'Zen Publications, Huddersfield

Pyves G 2001 'No hands' massage – squaring the circle of practitioner damage. Journal of Bodywork and Movement Therapies 5(3):173–180

Watson D 2000 An investigation into the links between massage practice and musculoskeletal damage to the practitioner's hands and wrists. Shi'Zen Publications, Huddersfield

USEFUL ADDRESS

Peter Mackereth and Gwynneth Campbell
The Rehabilitation Unit, Christie Hospital
Wilmslow Road
Manchester M20 4BX
UK
Tel: 0161 446 8236

Details of chair massage and other specialist training courses for therapists are available from Linda Orrett at the same address.

16

Being met with care: massage work with vulnerable patients

Nataly Lebouleux and Ann Carter

Abstract

This chapter explores the development and maintenance of the therapeutic relationship. The context in which the therapist works is described with the emphasis on working with vulnerable patients living with cancer. A reflective commentary has been incorporated from the principal author to examine core issues, for example being a facilitator rather than an expert. Recommendations are made identifying ways in which therapists can work sensitively with vulnerable individuals.

KEYWORDS

massage, vulnerability, relationship, expert, contract, context

INTRODUCTION

From the onset of a therapeutic relationship, any therapist can exert a certain amount of contextual power. Mitchell and Cormack (1998) believe that when a patient is in need, there is a potential loss of control; the patient accepts or defers to the perceived expertise of the health professional. Sometimes, a massage therapist may be perceived by patients as a nurse or physiotherapist who also provides massage. This is often not the case and changing perceptions of a therapist's role can be challenging for the patient. Massage therapists have an ethical responsibility to use their particular technical skills, expertise and time wisely, so that patients will not be physically or emotionally harmed. This is even more important as patients may feel vulnerable when they visit a massage therapist. The massage intervention should offer an empowering experience to an individual at all times. The work can help patients to identify or clarify what they need in terms of comfort and relaxation in the here and now. The intention of the work varies with the needs of the patients, although this may not always be explicit at the start of the treatment. Patients may not consciously know, or be able to articulate, what they need from the massage (Mackereth 2000). In maintaining a two-way process with patients, any therapist needs to adopt a facilitating role to achieve clarity in therapeutic work (Mitchell & Cormack 1998).

The emerging relationship between therapist and patient forms the main theme of this chapter. The components of this relationship include being aware of patient vulnerability, helping patients to receive what they need from massage, and using approaches which help individuals take back control. Key issues to be discussed are the context, the therapeutic contract, and being compassionate and present for others. Throughout the text the principal author makes reflective comments to illustrate how to work with concerns and issues in practice.

CONTEXTUAL ISSUES

Often, with a diagnosis of cancer, the journey is a bumpy one. Patients experience a roller coaster where moments of hope alternate with moments of despair, depending on the results from their latest scan or from surgery. When the results are not good, most patients undoubtedly experience a feeling of having been let down once more, this time by both their own bodies and the inability of drugs to cure the cancer. An encounter with a massage therapist may be the first time that a patient has met a therapist working differently from a conventional health professional. Being massaged is very different from the touch which can be experienced when being investigated, receiving surgery, chemotherapy and radiotherapy. Mitzi Blennerhassett has talked about her experience as a patient; Mitzi likened it to being on a production line, where one medical treatment was received after another. There was no real communication with healthcare professionals, she said she was 'floating in no-man's land' and wanted a 'hand to hold hers' (Blennerhassett 1996, p. 25).

Following introductions and a brief explanation of the therapy and how the treatment will be carried out, it is usual for the therapist to take a 'case history from the patient' as in any clinical practice. Care has to be taken not to engage the patient in a narrative of the cancer journey that is so complex and emotional that it inhibits a relaxing and nurturing experience. The purpose in receiving massage is to be touched in a therapeutic manner, with the 'how' and 'why' being a creative and uniquely individual process between the patient and therapist. Meeting 'in touch' can include technical skills and expertise the therapist has, the way the skills and expertise are applied together, and the way the therapist relates to the vulnerable patient within the therapeutic relationship.

Identifying a person's degree and state of vulnerability is complex and risks making judgements about an individual's ability to cope and exercise autonomy. Vulnerability has been defined as 'the state of being vulnerable, while the term "vulnerable" has been described as "able to be wounded" [of a person] ... able to be physically or emotionally hurt; liable to damage or harm especially from aggression or attack, assailable' (Concise Oxford Dictionary 1999). Massage could be construed as an assault if the patient has not fully consented (Stone 2002). Prior to, and during any touch-based intervention, it is essential ethical practice to ascertain that the patient has agreed and wishes to continue with the treatment. Power concerns in working with vulnerable patients have been raised by others working in hospice and cancer care. For example, Penson (1998) has acknowledged that patients may be compliant to unwanted treatments as a form of negotiation – if I am compliant, it will all be OK. There is a need for any therapist to ask themselves questions while working with patients who may be deemed vulnerable (see Box 16.1). It may also be useful for a therapist to seek supervisory support in examining the 'how' and 'why' of working with patients in this context (see Chapter 4).

Box 16.1
Power concerns in touch therapies

Therapists can reflect on their work using the following key questions:

- Who is in control of the treatment and what are the implications?
- Am I listening to the patient or pushing my own agenda?
- Am I truly supporting what the patient wants?
- How do I know I am working most appropriately with this patient?
- How can I give them choice?
- How can our work together offer opportunities for empowerment?

MASSAGE AS A POTENT INTERVENTION

When given a diagnosis of cancer many patients may feel they have no option but to accept chemotherapy, radiotherapy and/or surgery. Offering massage as a complementary therapy does provide a patient with, at least, the opportunity to give a 'No' or even a 'Well, maybe later' answer. Some patients may feel that they should say 'Yes' to everything available, particularly when a healthcare professional has made the referral. Patients may also view massage as something that will be done to them. It is important to differentiate between seeing patients as the passive recipients of the therapist's expertise in receiving treatment. Acknowledgement is required on both sides that the patient, although very ill, has knowledge and experience to contribute to the treatment. This understanding will develop and inform the work that takes place if therapist and patient work as a team, in mutual respect of each other's contribution. The relationship with patients works best when therapists can adjust their ways of practising, so that patients feel involved as partners in the process. Patients receiving a massage are on a learning curve, they may not know enough at the beginning of the massage process to contribute fully as a partner. The therapist needs to be open to this evolving role for the patient (Commentary 16.1).

Commentary 16.1

The therapist can offer techniques, sensitivity and a professional approach, that is without question. However, massage therapists cannot know in advance what patients will need and enjoy, and what they need to help them relax. This information can only be discovered if the therapist communicates with the patient. The massage therapist accepts that he or she has the skills and the sensitivity to help – this is but half of the story. The patient knows the other half, but that may not be apparent until later. It is helpful if the therapist is able to recognise and work with the concept that the patients are experts about their own body and what it needs.

There can be a choice, for example, in how a massage is received and experienced. When going through the different stages of having surgery, chemotherapy or radiotherapy treatment for cancer, patients may perceive that their body is like a machine that is failing and needs fixing. This interpretation is based on an assumption that there is a separation between body, mind, emotions and spirituality. In handing over the body for 'fixing', patients can become disconnected and anxious about how the body responds. When receiving massage, patients can learn to repossess their own physical selves, and adopt a mindset that the treatment will help their body to recover or ease symptoms. In restoring the balance, much of the work a massage therapist can do is to help the patient restore a greater sense of self.

Body image can be such a painful issue for many patients that they may perceive parts of themselves as 'an ugly thing'. Massage can offer 'containment for what has previously been experienced as uncontainable – unacceptable and unspeakable perception of a changed body and self' (Bredin 2001, p. 418). When the experience of massage is pleasurable (which it usually is), patients can begin to experience their physicality more positively, so they relate to their bodies rather as a new friend rather than an old adversary.

Massage treatments have been described by patients as 'soothing', 'comforting' and 'deeply relaxing'. This awakening experience of pleasure can counteract some of the pain and side effects associated with conventional medical treatments. Massage and touch therapies may not be life-saving, but quality of life, personal integrity and self-recognition of the patient as an individual can be enhanced. All of these components can help in reclaiming the body in a fuller sense, even at a late stage of illness, by appreciating pleasure and enjoyment in receiving a massage as healing experience (Bredin 2001).

CLARIFYING THE ROLE OF THE MASSAGE THERAPIST

In the era of evidence-based practice, massage outcomes are sometimes difficult to fully categorise. This means that exaggerated benefits are not expected by patients and/or cannot be claimed by therapists. This is both problematic but also advantageous. Mitchell and Cormack (1998) have argued that knowledgeable and skilful healthcare professionals are sometimes impossibly burdened with being viewed as all-knowing and perfect healers by patients. Recognition that this is not the case can 'free patients to find or use their own personal power, knowledge and strength' (p. 132). Massage could be judged to be both an art and a craft, but not a curative fix for cancer. Patients therefore may not have expectations of the massage beyond that of relaxation and enjoyment. However, patients can be surprised by the therapeutic benefits of massage, for example, in helping them sleep, reducing anxiety and maybe even feeling at ease and uplifted, despite the cancer. In identifying possible benefits, the therapist needs to explain that the intervention does not target one specific problem. Using a model for contracting with patients can be helpful in exploring how patients feel, what they would like, and any limitations to the work. Included within any contract is a basic ethical tenet, that of being able to say 'No', and at any point being able and supported to ask for the treatment to stop.

THE 'STOP, CLARIFY AND START AGAIN' CONTRACT

It is often too easy just to ask a patient to sit or lie down and have a massage treatment. Mackereth et al (2004) believe that an important part of the consent process is empowering the patient to stop the treatment, or to change the approach at any time. In palliative care, a therapist's intentions are to help. However, this can be experienced as rescuing, to the point that a patient feels that he or she must agree to whatever is offered. As discussed above, patients can be so disempowered by their illness that to be compliant with healthcare professionals may be an easier way of 'fitting in', or not appearing to be demanding. Pleasing others by acquiescing can be easier than saying, 'No, I don't want this right now'. It is therefore essential that while nine out of 10 people will be eager to receive a touch therapy, the therapist also needs to recognise and support the patient's right to decline touch at any point in offering and providing massage.

Agreeing that a patient can ask to stop the session and clarify the contract at any time could actually be tested in the first session. For example, a therapist could suggest that the patient actually stops the session verbally in the first few minutes and then asks for a change in the work. The change could be in repeating a movement, or working more gently or pausing for a moment. This could help to affirm the contract agreement that they can ask to change or stop the physical contact. Hunter and Struve (1998) recommend that therapists protect themselves and their patients by having a clear contract and consent for any touch in therapeutic work.

A MODEL FOR MASSAGE AND BODYWORK CONTRACTS

From experience, the authors have found that on most occasions patients are reluctant to express what they want from the treatment and are more likely to assume or expect the therapist to take responsibility for the massage, again believing the therapist knows best (see Commentary 16.2).

Commentary 16.2

When I ask patients, 'How would you like to feel by the end of the session?' or 'What would you like during the session?', they will often respond with, 'Do what you want with me. You know what's best' or 'Do what you think is best'. From the onset of the therapeutic relationship, patients will often place their bodies, and hence themselves, into the therapist's caring hands, willingly relinquishing their power, convinced that this is the only way to go.

Mackereth (2000) has devised the Structural, Emotional and Energetic Model for therapeutic contracts in reflexology, massage and bodywork to help establish a working contract with a patient wanting massage and bodywork (Box 16.2).

The model can be used to identify what the person's main reason is for coming for massage. A patient presenting with physical tension may have this symptom for a variety of reasons and it may not be appropriate to focus purely on releasing tight muscles (see Commentary 16.3). Exploring with the patient how he or she wants to work with the tension could start with the therapist asking, 'What's happening right now?' of the patient. It may be that the individual's response suggests that the therapist focuses on working at an emotional level, with holding techniques and witnessing the patient's concerns (see Commentary 16.3).

Commentary 16.3

Tensions are here for reasons that first need to be acknowledged. Sometimes, they are emotional, or postural, or they can simply be a way that someone had found to try and keep herself together in the face of adversity. Helping patients to realise why a tension is present can be empowering; once the tension is understood the patient may be able to do something about it. Massage, offered as the skilful use of touch, seems to provide patients with an opportunity to reclaim something. It is like discovering a lost kingdom ... their bodies!

> ## Box 16.2
> ## A model for massage and bodywork contracts: Structural, Emotional and Energetic (SEE)*
>
> ### Structural
>
> - Reduce muscle ache and tension, e.g. related to stress, postural problems.
> - Manage physical symptoms of anxiety, e.g. restlessness, insomnia.
> - Improve and support the cardiovascular system.
> - Support and maximise muscle function.
> - Help digestion and excretory functions.
> - Improve libido and sensuality.
> - Support for healing and prevention of illness.
> - Management of, and improve resistance to, stress.
>
> ### Emotional
>
> - Connect with feelings through/about the body.
> - Meet and contain potentially overwhelming emotions.
> - Witness, hold and comfort.
> - Nurture self-esteem and feelings of wellbeing.
> - Support process/personal development work.†
>
> ### Energetic‡
>
> - Acknowledgement and honouring of depletion of energy.
> - Open the body to restoring and holding energy.
> - Release energy that is blocked.
> - Connect synergistically with energy in a room/between the therapist and patient/using visualisation/colour/ritual/symbols.
> - Expansion beyond and encompassing the physical body.
> - Pleasurable energy moving through the body – 'joy unfolding'.
> - Strengthen energetic connection with the earth – 'grounding'.
>
> ---
>
> *Mackereth (2000).
> †This work would require the patient or carer to be in psychotherapy or counselling.
> ‡The term energy can be interpreted to mean chi, prana or other cultural and spiritual concepts of energy.

The awareness described in Commentary 16.3 can be surprising for many patients. It is as if massage offers a way of focusing their minds internally and acknowledging the sensations triggered by the massage as a 'feeling' map. Through following an internal sensory pathway, patients can learn ways of not 'being in their heads' but 'descending into their bodies'.

As patients learn to develop their own body awareness, they are able to discover new levels of relaxation and intimacy with themselves, and sometimes reach a state where the body is simply overwhelmed by a deep sense of peace or bliss. This can also be very soothing for clients who have to deal with physical pain and some patients described this state of simply 'being' as a spiritual experience (see Case study 16.1).

Case study 16.1

Christine, aged 34, had liver cancer and the therapist first treated her when she was in her last few weeks of life. Christine asked the therapist to use mainly caring, respectful touch in areas that she chose for herself at the beginning of the session. Christine used to describe her experience of very gentle massage as something 'spiritual', as if her body 'was not there, although it was there'. She found the treatment very soothing. It was a way of being with herself, and at the same time, beyond herself, which brought her peace and temporary relief from pain.

Box 16.3
Recommendations

- Therapists must acknowledge the ethical issues in working with patients who are living with cancer.
- Therapists must ensure that patients know that they can say 'No' to massage at any point during treatment.
- Therapists should ask themselves reflective questions and receive supervisory support to protect and safeguard the therapeutic relationship.
- The approach to techniques, contact and therapeutic skills needs adapting for individual patients.
- Therapists who wish to work with patients at levels other than the physical may need more in-depth training in working with emotions, body image issues and spiritual concerns.

SUMMARY

This chapter has examined the relationship between patient and massage therapist. Concerns such as vulnerability, control, body awareness and the therapeutic contract have been explored. Recommendations have been made in Box 16.3 to guide ethical, safe, and individualised massage practice.

REFERENCES

Bredin M 2001 Altered self-concept. In: Corner J, Bailey C (eds) Cancer nursing: care in context. Blackwell Science, Oxford

Blennerhassett M 1996 The pain of gentle touch. Health Service Journal 11 April, p. 25

Hunter M, Struve J 1998 The ethical use of touch in psychotherapy. Sage Publications, London

Mackereth P 2000 Tough places to be tender: contracting for happy or 'good enough' endings in therapeutic massage/bodywork? Complementary Therapies in Nursing and Midwifery 6(3):111–115

Mackereth P, Stringer J, Lynch B et al 2004 How CAM helps at acute cancer hospital. Journal of Holistic Health Care 1(1):33–38

Mitchell A, Cormack M 1998 The therapeutic relationship in complementary health care. Churchill Livingstone, London

Penson J 1998 Complementary therapies: making a difference in palliative care. Complementary Therapies in Nursing and Midwifery 4(3):77–81

Stone J 2002 Identifying ethicolegal and professional principles. In: Mackereth P, Tiran D (eds) Clinical reflexology: a guide for health professionals. Churchill Livingstone, Edinburgh

The Concise Oxford Dictionary, 10th edn. 1999 Oxford University Press, Oxford

FURTHER READING

Mitchell A, Cormack M 1998 The therapeutic relationship in complementary health care. Churchill Livingstone, London

USEFUL ADDRESS

Nataly Lebouleux
Therapeutic Massage Therapist
St Ann's Hospice
Neil Cliffe Cancer Care Centre
Wythenshawe Hospital
Southmoor Road
Wythenshawe
Manchester M23 9LT
UK
Tel: 0161 291 2912

Index

Training and expertise of therapists
(Continued)
  for research-consciousness, 38
  for safe adaptation of practice, 58–59
Transactional analysis
  ego states in therapeutic relationship,
    74–75
  recognition of being okay, 90
Transference, 72, 75, 89, 94–95
  counter-transference, 75, 89, 91, 94–95
  see also Somatic resonance
Trauma, 83, 180–181
  current trauma therapies, 97
  trauma/discharge model of body
    psychotherapy, 87
Tsubos ('gateways' in shiatsu), 158
Tumours, 5, 8–9, 11, 12, 108
  see also Cancer; Lymphoma; Myeloma

Unconscious mind, techniques for
    accessing, 79–80, 87
  nogotiation to work with, 76
Unsealed source therapy, 12

Visualisation, 22, 77, 79–80, 213
  see also Dream work; Guided imagery
Vollmer, H and Mills, D, 59
Vulnerability, 63, 74–75, 75–76, 107, 138,
    231–232

Wall, A, 105–106, 107
Wilkinson, S et al, 41, 47

Yin and yang, 159

Zen shiatsu, 157–161
  see also Shiatsu